PARKINSON'S DISEASE

DISEASE

The *New* Nutritional Handbook

A GUIDE FOR DOCTORS, NUTRITIONISTS, PATIENTS AND CARERS

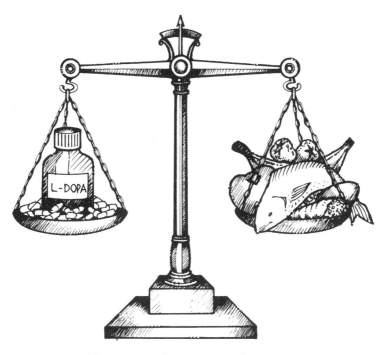

Dr. Geoffrey Leader MB.Ch.B. F.R.C.A.
Lucille Leader Dip. I.O.N.

ISBN   0 9526056 1 9

British Library Cataloguing in Publication Data. A catalogue record for this book is available from the British Library.

American Library of Congress Cataloguing in Publication Data

Printed in Great Britain by The Bath Press, Bath

Published in Great Britain in 1996 by Denor Press

PO. Box 12913, London N12 ONP

Cover Design by Fiona MacKenzie and CREATE, Bath, U.K.

DEDICATION

To Joe,
Erich, Karen, Esther and Ray

To people with Parkinson's Disease who wish to
optimise their health.

Special Acknowledgements

We wish to warmly thank the following people for their professional and
moral support during the preparation of this book:

Dr Erich Segal, Karen Segal, Janet Anders and Esther Orden for
proof reading and editing.

Dr Serena Leader-Morris and Rachel Leader for consultation.

Ashter Chomoko for book design and layout.

Fiona Mackenzie for cover artwork.

Veronica Nixon and Felicia Beder for secretarial and moral
support.

Joe Leader for annotated diagrams, computing and much patience.

Amir Gulamhusein of Highgate Stationers & Printers, London,
for assistance.

Brendan Beder, Robert Morris, Patricia and Morris Orden for
encouragement.

Last but not least, we wish to acknowledge Dr Herman Hagens
who originally inspired our interest in applied biochemistry
which forms the basis of modern clinical nutrition.

DR GEOFFREY L LEADER M.B., CH.B., F.R.C.A.

Geoffrey Leader is a Consultant Anaesthetist and Medical Director of The London Pain Relief and Nutritional Support Clinic at the Devonshire Hospital in London. He is particularly interested in the nutritional support of patients with chronic illness.

Dr Leader is a Fellow of the Royal College of Anaesthestists and has worked as a Consultant Anaesthetist as Head of Departments at University Hospitals in The Netherlands, South Africa and in London. He has published papers on long-term naso-tracheal intubation in neonates and the use of the laryngeal mask during facial surgery.

Geoffrey Leader's last academic post was: Chairman of the Anaesthetic Department, Honorary Senior Consultant, Senior Lecturer, Head of Intensive Care and Pain Clinic at Newham General Hospital. This Unit forms part of the Royal London Hospital Medical College, University of London. He is now in Private Practice in London, his specialist fields being Anaesthesia, the Nutritional Support of chronically ill patients and Pain Relief. He is involved in research in the field of Parkinson's Disease.

LUCILLE LEADER DIP. I.O.N.

Lucille Leader is a nutritionist who is particularly interested in the nutritional needs of people with chronic illness.

She works in association with Dr. Geoffrey Leader, M.B., Ch.B., F.R.C.A., her husband, whose specialist fields are Anaesthesia, Chronic Pain Relief and Nutrition. They practice at the Devonshire Hospital in London, England.

Her late father, Dr. Joseph Orden, was particularly interested in the role of nutrition in preventive medicine.

She has completed a research project entitled "Analysis of the Effects of the Removal of the Gluten and other Unknown Compounds contained in Wheat and Gluten Grains, Rye, Oats and Barley in Sufferers of the Irritable Bowel Syndrome," under Dr Philip Barlow, M.Sc., Ph.D., Dean of the School of Applied Science and Technology, University of Humberside and Supervisor of Research Projects at The Institute for Optimum Nutrition in London. She is also involved in research in the field of Parkinson's Disease.

The nutritional protocols described in this book are used at their Clinic by Dr Geoffrey Leader and Lucille Leader. She is also very interested in the nutritional management of Inflammatory Diseases.

CONTENTS

INTRODUCTION BY THE AUTHORS 1

PART 1   7

1.1. NUTRITIONAL BIOCHEMICAL APPROACH 9
   Biochemical Tests 10
   Supplements of Vitamins, Minerals, Essential Fatty Acids and Free
   Form Amino Acids whether Patients use Medication or Not 11
   Suggested Basic Supplemental Nutrient Cover 12
   Diet (The Raw Materials) and the Parkinson's Patient 13
   Diet (A Simplified 'Biochemical' Approach) 13
   Conclusion 17

**1.2. THE NUTRITIONAL MANAGEMENT OF PATIENTS
WITH PARKINSON'S DISEASE WHO ARE RELIANT ON L-DOPA
MEDICATION** 18
   Discussion 19

**1.3. FOOD FACTS - FOR PATIENTS USING PHARMACEUTICAL L-DOPA
(PROBLEMS AND SOLUTIONS)** 20
   Protein 20
   Dairy Foods 21
   Grains 21
   Nuts, Seeds and Pulses 22
   Stimulants (Alcohol, Tea, Coffee, Chocolate) 23
   Yeast 23
   Balancing Blood Sugar Levels 24

1.4. FOODS COMPATIBLE WITH THE ABSORPTION OF LEVODOPA 25
   Grains 25
   Vegetables 25
   Oils 25
   Herb Teas 25
   Coffee Substitutes 26
   Water 26
   Spreads 26
   Breads, Biscuits and Cakes 26

Fruit 26
Fruit Juices 27
Milk Substitutes 27
Social Drinks 27
Vegetable Stock Cubes Or Powders (Bouillon Cubes) 27

1.5. HIGH PROPORTION PROTEIN FOODS FOR THE
"PROTEIN WINDOW PERIOD" ONLY 28
Proteins Containing Essential Amino Acids: 28

1.6. CONSTIPATION 29

1.7. A PRACTICAL METHOD FOR ALLEVIATING CONSTIPATION 31

1.8. FIBRE-CONTAINING FOODS 34

1.9. STRESS AND DEPRESSION 35

1.10. PRACTICAL EATING SOLUTIONS 37
Sublingual, Transdermal, Intravenous and Oral Routes 38

1.11. NUTRITIONAL MANAGEMENT OF PATIENTS UNDERGOING
ANAESTHESIA WHO ARE RELIANT ON L-DOPA MEDICATION 39

PART 2   41

2.1. HOW NUTRITION INFLUENCES YOUR BODY 43
How the Body Makes its Own L-dopa and Dopamine 43
How Cells Make Energy in order to Carry Out their functions 44

2.2. SPECIAL PROBLEMS 45

2.3. DIET FOR THE PARKINSON'S PATIENT WHO IS
NOT ON L-DOPA MEDICATION 46

2.4. HOW TO USE AND UNDERSTAND THE DIET FOR USERS OF L-DOPA 48
Example 49
Choices and Preparation 49

2.5. LIST OF 'GOOD' FOOD TYPES 53
Carbohydrates 53
Fats 54
Proteins 54

2.6. ALTERNATIVE FOODS TO USE WHEN NEEDING THE
EFFECTS OF L-DOPA 55

2.7. ESSENTIAL PRACTICAL ADVICE **58**

2.8. RECIPES FOR GENERAL USE INCLUDING THE L-DOPA PERIOD **60**
Soups 60
Salads and Salad Dressings..63
Vegetarian Grain Recipes (Gluten Free and Low Protein)................65
Potato Delights..69
Cakes Biscuits and Pastry 71
Desserts 73

2.9. CONCENTRATED PROTEIN RECIPES **76**
Main meals..76
Puddings..77
Special Treats..78

2.10. NUTRIENT CONTENT OF BASIC FOODS....................................**79**
Calories, Quantity and Quality of Food...79
Some Good Food Sources of Nutrients..79

**2.11. SOME APPROXIMATE FOOD VALUES - MACRONUTRIENTS AND
CALORIES OF KEY CARBOHYDRATES, PROTEINS AND FATS** **85**
Carbohydrates 85
Proteins..86
Fats 87

APPENDIX   89

3.1. GLOSSARY OF TERMS **91**

3.2. REFERENCES..**96**

3.3. BIBLIOGRAPHY **99**

3.4. INDEX...**102**

DIAGRAMS

THE L-DOPA PATHWAYS 6
ATP (ENERGY) PRODUCTION AND THE KREBS CYCLE 8
SIX DIVISIONS OF THE BRAIN 40
A CELL 42

INTRODUCTION BY THE AUTHORS

As you no doubt know, people with Parkinson's Disease often present primarily with the symptoms of tremor, rigidity, unsteadiness and bradykinesia (slow movement). Consequently, various other related physiological and psychological problems occur. The reason for impaired muscle control seems to be due to a lack of the neurotransmitter, dopamine. Dopamine is manufactured by neurones in the substantia nigra area of the brain. These neurones may not produce sufficient dopamine due possibly to different reasons - precursor problems, degeneration, mitochondrial inadequacy, non-functioning enzymes, deficient cellular nutrition, cell death, disease, free radical destruction, environmental toxicity, drugs, genes. Current treatment is mainly based on the use of pharmaceutical medication, levodopa, (the precursor of dopamine) as well as dopamine agonists. Pallidotomy and foetal brain cell transplants are operative procedures being tried in a few centres internationally.

We are inspired to publish this programme for two reasons: in clinical practice, we come across needless suffering on the part of patients with Parkinson's Disease who take L-dopa medication - suffering associated with a "complex" of being "afraid to eat." This is because their symptoms related to muscular control sometimes worsen as a result. The effect of ingested L-dopa medication has somehow been undermined by the food. Patients sometimes unwittingly ingest complete or concentrated proteins during the precise times when they will compete with their medication for absorption. For this very reason the effects of their medication are impaired.

This inevitably leads to a host of physiological, biochemical and psychological problems. Patients are unable to fuel their bodies adequately with calories, vital carbohydrates, essential fats and protein (the essential amino acids which are phenylalanine, tryptophan, leucine, isoleucine, lycine, methionine, valine, threonine) vitamins and minerals which are necessary for basic energy and health maintenance. This could be quite apart from their dopamine related problems - which problem at this present time is addressed by taking medication providing levodopa (L-dopa). This leads to chronic fatigue and the unhealthy need for stimulants (tea, coffee, chocolate, alcohol and simple sugars) resulting in insomnia and added stress

1

due to unstable glycaemic (blood sugar) patterns. Weight loss, constipation and despair seem to be the order of the day, in addition to the possible onset of other illnesses due to inadequate cellular nutrition.

Secondly, in patients who do not take pharmaceutical L-dopa, we find a very poor general health status, chronic intractible constipation and multiple nutritional deficiencies including those nutrients which are essential and pertinent to the biosynthesis of neurotransmitters in addition to other biochemical functions.

However, one must bear in mind that there is a biochemical interrelation of all nutrients. The biosynthesis and efficacy of natural L-dopa in the substantia nigra, striatum and the adrenal medulla, requires balanced levels of acetylcholine, tyrosine, serotonin, vitamin C, vitamin B6 (pyridoxine phosphate) and glucose, the raw materials of which are found in food. One can therefore appreciate the importance of the choice of food to create optimum biochemical function. As some factors cannot be synthesised by the body, they are exclusively nutritionally based and are as such deemed essential. Examples are those amino acids which are converted into tyrosine and serotonin as well as vitamin C. Essential fatty acids, which contribute to the integrity of cellular membranes and the production of prostaglandins, also require dietary input for their synthesis.

Judging from the reports correlated from patients about their eating and drinking habits, we realised that there was an extra dimension common to the biochemical individuality of each and every person taking L-dopa supplementation. This was the competition for the absorption sites in the proximal small bowel as well as competition for active transport across the blood-brain barrier of most of the neutral amino acids (constituents of whole protein foods) with the drugs containing L-dopa. *(1,2)*.

It became obvious that there was a need for professional specialised nutritional guidance for people needing pharmaceutical L-dopa. In this programme total nutritional consideration was taken into account with recommendations for biochemical baselines. The delicious diet recommended is rational and ensures the optimal absorption of levodopa, together with all other essential nutrients and adequate calories. It is also suited to patients who do not take L-dopa medication. It provides for a healthy intestinal tract kept free for maximum absorption of levodopa and nutrients.

Foods are recommended which increase cellular energy, containing complex carbohydrates, vitamins and minerals needed in the Krebs Cycle. Food sources of L-dopa are mentioned as well as the recent introduction of NADH as a supplement for cellular energy. Fibre (soluble and insoluble), fluids and essential fatty acids are advised. The importance of efficacious digestive enzymes, the integrity of the gut wall and the presence of "friendly" Bifidobacteria in the intestine are also discussed. These aspects are vital to adequate absorption. Alleviation of constipation is also handled, as this is vital to the health of the intestinal tract.

The key to the management of the programme for users of L-dopa is knowing which foods are implicated in competing with levodopa and eliminating these around the time that L-dopa needs to be metabolised and absorbed. It is also knowing which foods can and should be ingested at that time in order to avoid malnutrition.

A full spectrum of pre-digested free form amino acids is also suggested during the period that levodopa is not being absorbed from the gut (most usually at night if the patient is taking L-dopa supplementation during the day.) It is fascinating to learn that the amino acid phenylalanine, broken down from protein, not only enters the dopamine pathway but also that of thyroxine, necessary for thyroid function as well. It also forms melanin. In addition, one sees that adrenalin (epinephrine) and noradrenalin (norepenephrine) *(7)* are processed from this same phenylalanine in the adrenal medulla.

In patients with Parkinson's Disease, whether they take L-dopa or not, biochemical testing may show deficiencies in amino acids, essential to the manufacture of neurotransmitters and other anabolic functions. Thyroid and adrenal function may also benefit from support bearing in mind that thyroxine is a metabolite of tyrosine *(3)*. Vitamins may also be deficient, particularly B vitamins which serve cellular energy (ATP) produced during the Krebs Cycle *(4,5)*. Vitamin B6, vital to the body's protein metabolism (in the form of pyridoxal phosphate) is a coenzyme to dihydroxy phenylalanine (dopa) decarboxylase, one of the 3 enzymes required for the formation of noradrenalin and results in dopamine being taken up into membranous vesicles, and the pathway for the biosynthesis of dopamine *(6)*. Essential fatty acids (Omega 6 and Omega 3) and antioxidant profiles could be lacking. These are essential for immune control and the integrity

3

of cellular membranes. All deficiencies should be addressed. Guidelines for biochemical testing, as well as nutritional supplementation are presented in this book.

Various topics are presented. Should patients be at a stage when they are unable to take food orally, feeds given by naso-gastric tube, feeding by tube directly into the stomach or intravenous feeding are recommended. Intravenous therapy is presented as it offers vital support to metabolism. Supplemental feeds should be chosen with an awareness of the protein content in these specially prepared liquids. The same principle which governs the choice of a specialised optimal diet for Parkinson's patients taking L-dopa medication should be exercised so as not to compromise its maximum absorption. This principle is the cornerstone of the nutritional programme for those reliant on pharmaceutical L-dopa.

Included are guidelines for stress management, practical solutions to eating problems, tips for safety in the kitchen and simple recipes for daily as well as social use. These recipes are based on the principles of maximisation of absorption of pharmaceutical L-dopa. Patients who do not take L-dopa can use these recipes too but they may eat any food type whenever they wish as there is no drug-nutrient interaction for them. Nonetheless they are made aware that wheat and dairy products are common allergens. They too are advised of other physiological, psychological and practical aids. It should be stated to all patients, however, that there are possible drug-nutrient reactions with any medication. This should be checked by contacting the technical information officer of the relevant drug manufacturer. Food values and calorie counters are also presented.

It is hoped that by following the recommendations in the book, a feeling of improved well-being, a better weight maintenance, help with constipation and tremor as a result of drug nutrient interaction may be achieved. Repetition of vital information appears intentionally at various sites in the book, which could be helpful for study purposes.

Dr P. Kempster MD, MRCP, FRACP and Professor M.L. Wahlqvist, MD, FRACP in Australia wrote recently in Nutrition Reviews *(8)*:

"The 20th century has seen the progressive development of the scientific basis of an expanding discipline of clinical nutrition, scarcely articulated until recently,".. (it can) "modulate the expression of disease and provide opportunities for management."

In August 1995, Peter Hayes, Consultant at The Royal Infirmary of Edinburgh, reviewing the book "Artificial Nutrition Support in Clinical Practice", wrote:

"...Clinical nutrition is an important and expanding area of medicine..." *(9)*.

Also, centuries ago, Hippocrates, the so-called "Father of Medicine" said: "Let food be your medicine" - and in this case, we sincerely hope that it will be!

Dr Geoffrey Leader and Lucille Leader

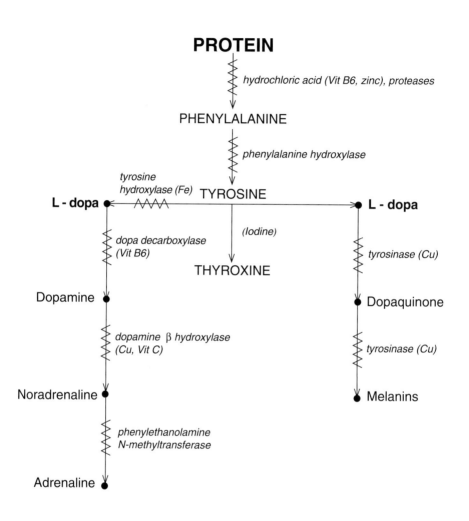

PROTEIN

hydrochloric acid (Vit B6, zinc), proteases

PHENYLALANINE

phenylalanine hydroxylase

tyrosine
hydroxylase (Fe) **TYROSINE**

L - dopa ••••••• **L - dopa**

dopa decarboxylase
(Vit B6)

(Iodine)

tyrosinase (Cu)

THYROXINE

Dopamine •   • Dopaquinone

dopamine β hydroxylase
(Cu, Vit C)

tyrosinase (Cu)

Noradrenaline •   • Melanins

phenylethanolamine
N-methyltransferase

Adrenaline •

The L- dopa pathways.

PART 1

Part 1 combines biochemical and technical information with practical recommendations.

Part 2 is specifically designed for the non-scientific reader and starts on page 41. It is user friendly and very easy to follow, meeting both practical and nutritional needs.

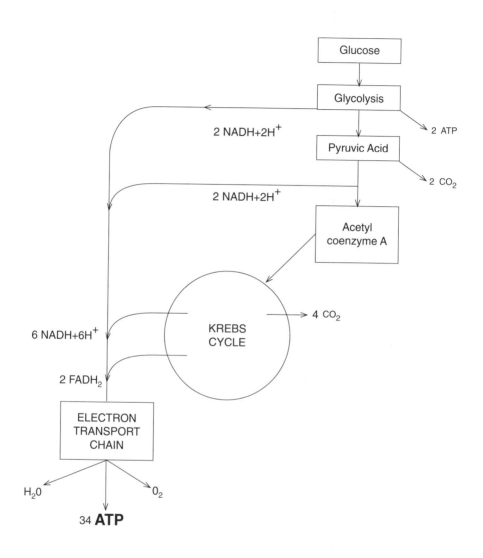

Production of ATP (energy) from glucose in the mitochondria. A summary

1.1. Nutritional Biochemical Approach

Optimum functional health is the goal of a specialist nutritional programme. In order to support this brief the cellular needs of each individual should be biochemically and clinically assessed for an orthomolecular approach to be calculated.

Mitochondria are the power house of the cell and current thinking suggests that mitochondrial exhaustion may be implicated in poor cellular function. Nutrition could aid in providing the raw material, precursors, co-enzymes and co-factors for the manufacture of ATP (cellular energy) in the Krebs Cycle. For example, carbohydrate, coenzyme Q10, coenzyme 1 (NADH), iron, biotin, B vitamins, magnesium and manganese, are amongst other nutrients, necessary for this biochemical process. NADH, a vital step in the making of ATP, is now available as a supplement and is being used by some with promising results *(10)*. It is known as coenzyme 1.

However, all cellular ingredients necessary to life's biochemical processes must be present in adequate supply for cellular energy to be able to be produced. Protein providing the essential amino acids pertinent to neurological and other anabolic activity, if deficient, should be addressed. Thyroid and adrenal functions should be monitored. Essential fatty acids pertinent to cell membrane integrity and prostaglandins should be present in sufficiency. Carbohydrates crucial to the glycaemic pathways as well as vital vitamins and minerals which play their roles in the body's biochemical processes, should be adequately present. Antioxidant nutrients are necessary for the control of free radicals. General nutritional status may therefore contribute to the enhancement of general function and energy in the Parkinson's patient.

The inability of cells to detoxify at an adequate rate relative to intoxication is also under consideration these days. Strategies to lighten the load of toxins to which the human body is exposed - environmental (such as radiation, organophosphates, lead, mercury), nutritional (for example food additives, micro-organisms), chemical (drugs) could be helpful. Optimising the bodily functions of elimination - breathing, passing of urine and bowel movements, as well as the use of chelating agents could be of help in maintenance of functional health. There might well be an indication for detoxification as well as chelation therapy.

Good Digestive potential (enzymes), as well as effective absorptive capabilities (status of the intestinal wall) in patients are the underlying requirements for optimum cellular potential. If this is not the case, remedial therapy should be instigated as an alternative to oral feeding or supplemental to it. (Tube and intravenous nutritional therapy.)

The Parkinson's patient surely deserves to function as best as he potentially can on all levels. With the addressing of deficiencies which are vital to the body's general biochemical needs, the biosynthesis of neurotransmitters, cellular energy (ATP), integrity of cell membranes and the control of free radical damage, it could perhaps be hypothetically possible for patients to find that they require less pharmaceutical support generally. This could also possibly apply to a reduction in the amount of pharmaceutical L-dopa being taken, provided that there are still sufficient neurones able to function. Should this be possible, it could be postulated that those neurones might then be able to produce their own neurotransmitters. Feedback mechanisms which had long since ceased to function because the synthesis of L-dopa had been taken over completely for them, could possibly be re-instated. Certainly the experience of the Birkmeyer Clinic for PD Therapy in Vienna is that with their use of NADH which stimulates the synthesis of ATP, in certain cases, phamaceutical L-dopa is able to be reduced *(11)*. NADH could also be useful in stimulating the production of cellular energy in patients who are not on L-dopa.

There has been research done on the efficacy of food containing L-dopa (Vicia faba broad beans)*(12)*. Certainly other foods provide the raw materials necessary for physiological and biochemical activity, providing that digestion and absorption function adequately.

Biochemical Tests

For the individuality of patients whether using medication or not

In addition to routine Haematology, Biochemistry and Thyroid Function tests, it is useful to test for the status of vitamins, minerals, essential fatty acids, amino acids and antioxidant profiles in patients. Helicobacter and other parasitic assays may be indicated as well as urinalysis.

Digestive enzyme potential and Gut Permeability should also be checked, so that a specialised nutritional programme may be drawn up based on the biochemical individuality of each patient. IgE and IgG Tests could help identify allergy or intolerance. Even IgA testing can be useful. The Adrenal

Stress Indicator Test is a useful indicator for therapy. Screening for toxicity, for example, mercury, cadmium and lead should be performed. Exposure to organophosphates and organochlorine compounds should be monitored.

Cardio-vascular screening should be considered in order to exclude any significant decrease in cerebral circulation as this might influence the efficacy of medication.

Base line tests such as those outlined in this section are extremely useful in designing a therapeutic nutritional support programme for Parkinson's sufferers. Due to their inadequate nutritional patterns, free radical damage, use of strong laxatives, stress and imbibement of dietary stimulants, their basic cellular nutritional status which is necessary for optimal function, is often deficient. Any inflammation or candidiasis perhaps due to frequent use of antibiotics and which could possibly potentiate a dysbiosis of gut flora should be assessed. This is needed to design an approach for optimal intestinal function.

Note: Specialised nutritional tests including gastrogram (for assessing digestive enzymes), gut fermentation, gut permeability, nutrient profiles for vitamins, minerals and essential fatty acids, IgE, IgG and IgA are available *(13)*.

Supplements of Vitamins, Minerals, Essential Fatty Acids and Free Form Amino Acids whether Patients use Medication or Not

Food And Nutrients
As food today frequently offers reduced nutritional value due to inadequate soil or long shelf life, the goal of achieving a healthy balanced diet is becoming a myth. It might well be advisable to supplement basic levels of vitamins, minerals, essential fatty acids (omega 3 and omega 6) and a full spectrum of pre-digested free form amino acids for general health maintenance, apart from "therapeutic doses", as indicated biochemically.

Note for Patients on L-dopa medication: any amino acid therapy as well as the essential fatty acids (which contain amino acids) should only occur during the "protein window period," as they contain concentrated protein and will compete for absorption with L-dopa.

Suggested Basic Supplemental Nutrient Cover

(Free from wheat, gluten, dairy, colour and chemical preservative. Most bioavailable forms or sublinguals should be considered.)

- General vitamins (A, C, E, D, B complex)
- B complex (containing vitamin B6 preferably in the form of pyridoxal 5 phosphate) may be taken with Sinemet *(14)* and Madopar products because of the administration of a peripheral decarboxylase inhibitor within the medication.) B3 may sometimes cause flushing and discomfort because of vasodilation. The health professional must gauge the dose accordingly. It is necessary to administer adequate zinc together with vitamin B6 (pyridoxal 5 phosphate).
- Vitamin C is best taken as magnesium ascorbate, to avoid acidity
- Biotin
- Folic acid
- Minerals - organic forms (containing at least 15mg elemental value of zinc as a citrate or amino-acid chelate, magnesium EAP, calcium EAP, boron, manganese, chromium, polynicotinate for the support of glucose tolerance factor, iron if indicated, molybdenum, selenium.)
- Omega 6 essential fatty acids (GLA),
- Omega 3 essential fatty acids (EPA)
- Full spectrum of free form predigested amino acids (during "protein window period").
- Acetylcholine or lecithin granules
- Antioxidant formula
- Acidophilus Bifido bacteria (Probiotics) *(15,16)*.
- Coenzyme Q10 (lipid formulation)
- Coenzyme 1 (NADH)
- Digestive enzymes if indicated
- Valerian if indicated for tranquilisation
- Suitable formulation for liver support or detox
- Formulations to assist in the healing of gut hyperpermeability if indicated. They should optimally contain L-glutamine

IMPORTANT NOTE

Vitamins, minerals and NADH may be given intravenously as a booster at the initiation of the supplement programme or if the patient is malabsorbing.

Diet (The Raw Materials) and the Parkinson's Patient

(whether using L-dopa Medication or not)

During a 24-hour period, complex carbohydrates, complete proteins containing the essential amino acids, essential fatty acids, foods containing vital minerals and vitamins as well as sufficient fluids should be consumed.

Fruits, vegetables, grains (non-gluten), still mineral water, juices diluted with water, herb teas and vegetable type coffee drinks may be enjoyed. Sea fish, white flesh of poultry and pulses may be eaten. Caffeine, alcohol and refined sugars are to be avoided. (Attention should be paid to sufficient appropriate fibre (gluten-free) and adequate fluids to assist with peristalsis.)

Patients not on L-dopa medication may eat proteins freely, but those using L-dopa medication should only take protein foods or amino-acid supplements well away from medication time.

Diet (A Simplified 'Biochemical' Approach)

(Lists of nutrient contents of foods are to be found in Part 2)

It is food that provides the body with the raw materials necessary for life's essential functions. If digestive enzymes are sufficient, these raw materials - proteins, carbohydrates and fats - carrying vitamins and minerals, are broken down from larger molecules into small forms usable and acceptable to the system. If the intestinal wall is in good condition (for example, not hyperpermeable, inflamed or ulcerated), these "broken down", fully digested molecules will be absorbed effectively through it into the bloodstream and carried via the liver (for detoxification and/or storage) to eventually all cells of the body. There they will be stored or metabolized to provide the necessary services to the function of that particular cell.

One realises that optimal intestinal health is crucial to adequate digestion and absorption of vital nutrients.

A good diet must include protein, carbohyrates, fats, vitamins, minerals and water. This is the stuff of which human beings are made! The following condensed resume of just a few functions of these essential raw materials in the body should suffice to motivate the reader as to the importance of the regular choice of suitable foods and the vital need for supporting the integrity of the gastro-intestinal tract.

Proteins

Under the influence of hydrochloric acid, zinc, vitamin B6 and proteases, proteins break down into amino acids before being absorbed into the blood stream for distribution to cells. There are 8 essential amino acids which are necessary to life but as the body cannot synthesise them, they are only available in what is eaten. Foods which contain them are complete or whole proteins such as eggs, fish, meat and soya beans. Certain other foods may also be combined which together make up the eight essential fatty acids (each food item may contain some, but not all, of the required eight.)

Amino acids are involved in anabolic cellular processes. Of particular interest to patients with Parkinson's Disease is the fact that certain amino acids are directly responsible for the efficacy of dopamine in the brain as well as in the adrenal medulla. These are tryptophan and phenylalanine. Thereafter these become respectively the neurotransmitters serotonin and dopamine. The right balance between these materials and acetylcholine must exist - otherwise their interaction may possibly cause over or under stimulation of neurones. This could result in impaired motor control as is found in Parkinson's Disease *(17)*.

Acetylcholine

This is a neurotransmitter made from choline found, for example, in the protein foods fish and soya lecithin. Pantothenic acid (vitamin B5) is required for the conversion from choline to acetylcholine in the brain. It affects the emotions of sex and plays a role in memory and learning. Deficiency can cause decreased concentration, sleeplessness and poor muscle coordination. Mucus membranes necessary for the activity of acetylcholine become dry and easily susceptible to irritation and infection *(18)*. Support for the membranes using nutrients that contain the essential fatty acids and anti-oxidants which are a support against free radical activity, could be helpful.

Tryptophan

Tryptophan is an essential amino acid used by the brain to make the neurotransmitter serotonin. It can be found in milk and bananas. Deficiency results in sleep disorders and is often seen in the elderly.

Phenylalanine

Tyrosine evolves from the essential amino acid, phenylalanine, found in protein foods such as eggs, cheese, meat and nuts. Dopamine is made from tyrosine. An enzyme, tyrosine hydroxylase, converts tyrosine into a chemical called levodopa. This levodopa (L-dopa) is then converted into dopamine by another enzyme, dopa decarboxylase, which is dependent upon pyridoxal phosphate (vitamin B6) as a co-enzyme *(19)*. ATP, cellular energy, produced during the Krebs Cycle, is dependent on glucose, B vitamins, vitamin C, coenzyme Q10, coenzyme 1, iron, copper, oxygen, magnesium, manganese and biotin, and accompanies these processes *(20)*.

All these factors necessary for the biochemical processing of tyrosine are to be found in foods. There are food lists in *Part 2* of this book citing sources of nutrients.

It is fascinating to note that phenylalanine, after being synthesized into tyrosine, can also become thyroxine for thyroid function as well as adrenalin (epenephrine) and noradrenalin (norepenephrine) for the adrenal medulla. Melanin in skin pigment is synthesised from tyrosine. Copper is necessary for this pathway. The implications to health are significant if there are problems arising from improper metabolic handling of tyrosine.

Carbohydrates
These are ideally eaten as complex carbohydrates, as found in grains such as brown rice, plantains, buckwheat, wholemeal wheat, whole rye and millet. They break down into glucose in the digestive tract, under the influence of digestive enzymes. This is absorbed through the gut wall into the blood stream and is carried to each cell where it forms the basis for the manufacture of cell energy - ATP. In order to do this satisfactorily B vitamins, vitamin C, magnesium, manganese, biotin, coenzyme Q10, coenzyme 1, iron and oxygen must be present. Lists in *Part 2* cite food sources of nutrients. It has been observed that the effect of oral L-dopa is improved by glucose loading *(21)*.

Various compartments of the brain need glucose and when this is not available and glycogen stores have been used up, ketone bodies are used by the brain as an energy-yielding substrate. This is not ideal, because other processes in the brain have a real need for glucose and ketones are not suitable in these cases. These processes may include the synthesis, in certain areas of the brain, of the ionotrophic neurotransmitters, such as acetylcholine *(22)*.

15

Fats

Certain vital fats known as the essential fatty acids (omega 6 and omega 3) are unable to be synthesised by the body and must be provided by food. They are to be found in cold pressed polyunsaturated oils such as linseed oil and evening primrose oil. Oleic acid is found in olives and is monounsaturated. The essential fatty acids are implicated in prostaglandin function which includes control of inflammation, support of cardiovascular disease and the integrity of cellular membranes, amongst other functions. See food lists in *Part 2*.

Vitamins

These are biochemical necessities as co-factors and co-enzymes in the body. If certain of them are deficient they can reduce cellular energy. Some pave the way for degenerative disease - for example, vitamin C and scurvy. Ascorbate is necessary in the enzyme dopamine B-hydroxylase which makes dopamine in the adrenal medulla. Vitamin B3 deficiency causes pellagra. Some are also involved in the biosynthesis of neurotransmitters in the brain, for example - pyridoxal phosphate (vitamin B6). Lists of foods containing vitamins are to be found in *Part 2*.

Minerals

These are biochemically necessary as co-factors and co-enzymes. Calcium, magnesium, phosphorus and boron are necessary for bone integrity, dependent upon Vitamin D3 for their absorption. Zinc is implicated in the activity of enzymes as well as male and female fertility, protein synthesis and a host of other biochemical necessities. It is also a chelator of toxic metals such as aluminium and lead. Iron is necessary for the manufacture of red blood cells and together with magnesium and manganese, is implicated in the Krebs Cycle during the manufacture of energy. Tyrosine hydroxylase, the rate limiting step in catecholemine synthesis, is iron dependant. Dopamine B-hydroxylase contains copper. Chromium is important to glucose tolerance factor and the enhancement of the action of insulin. Lists of foods containing minerals are to be found in *Part 2* of this book.

Food Sources Of L-dopa

There are vegetables which contain L-dopa in free-form (*23*). How these may be incorporated into the diet of patients reliant on the use of pharmaceutical L-dopa is best calculated by a health professional.

Conclusion

It is therefore obvious that a good diet should contain the raw materials necessary for the biosynthesis of all the body's basic requirements in order to support its cellular functions. However, ingestion does not necessarily mean proper digestion and absorption. The presence of adequate levels of digestive enzymes is essential, as is a healthy intestinal wall and a symbiosis of gut flora. Enzymes necessary for the biosynthesis of nutrients up to their final stages are also vital. The ability to chew and swallow must also be possible. These aspects must be assessed before health professionals can rely on the oral route. Otherwise it may be necessary to support the body by supplemental feeding of a specialised nature such as parenteral, sublingual, transdermal, via naso-gastric tube or feeding directly into the stomach. This could be whilst therapy is instigated to restore the integrity of the digestive tract or whilst patients are being stabilised on their drug regime.

Therapy using NADH, also called coenzyme 1, a vital stage in the manufacture of cellular energy, has been used by Professors Jorg and Walter Birkmeyer of The Birkmeyer Institute For PD Therapy in Vienna, Austria *(24)*.

Oral NADH is also known as reduced NAD. It is not the ordinary NAD sold in Health Shops. Its use must be supervised by a medical practitioner as doses of pharmaceutical L-dopa might need to be lowered, stopped or adjusted. Taking a lot of pharmaceutical L-dopa as well as NADH can result in hyperactivity and increase in muscular movements. It seems that NADH may increase the production of dopamine *(25.)* Other dietary factors and supplementation (given orally or boosted by intravenous therapy) which contribute the ingredients crucial to the Krebs Cycle should be available. NADH is a vital step in the last stage of the manufacture of cellular energy.

Antioxidants protect cellular membranes and could be helpful against free radical activity and should therefore be considered as part of nutritional support.

1.2. The Nutritional Management of Patients with Parkinson's Disease who are Reliant on L-dopa Medication

The key to successful food management in patients on L-dopa lies:

1. in their knowledge of which foods "compete" with L-dopa for absorption sites in the proximal small bowel

2. in their knowledge of which foods are available and are "compatible" with the optimum absorption of levodopa

3. in their imbibement of sufficient fluids, "appropriate fibre" and exercise to stimulate peristalsis as constipation could be a problem to patients

4. in their utilisation of a specific "protein window period" - the longest time during a 24 hour cycle in which the patient is not taking levodopa - to use this period to ingest concentrated protein essential to the maintenance of optimum health, which has had to be excluded during the rest of the day. (The exclusion of this in the diet, having been due to its competition with levodopa - the latter having been the most necessary substance for the body at that time)

5. in the maintenance of the integrity of the intestinal wall, thus ensuring "adequate absorption". To this end, the status of the digestive enzymes, the permeability of the intestinal wall and the adequacy of the intestinal flora should be assessed and treated if necessary

6. in the understanding that should complete feeding be indicated via tube, the "choice of feed should be either carbohydrate or protein based", depending on the times of administration of levodopa. This is to ensure that the amino acid content of the feed will not compete for the absorption sites which coincide with those of L-dopa in the proximal small bowel.

7. in a "diet" suited to optimum health using nutritional supplements.

8. in the use of "biochemical testing" to devise a nutritional programme based on individual biochemical individuality.

Discussion

The time of "kick-in" will commence depending on the type of pharmaceutical L-dopa taken (controlled or instant release). This could also vary with biochemical and physiological individuality.

It would therefore be advisable to assess the rate of gastric emptying in individual patients in order to work out what their optimum levodopa and feeding patterns should be.

Fasted or fed states with the ingestion of the medication should be assessed in each individual. This also depends on the type of medication taken. For instance, Madopar may be taken with food and Sinemet taken without.

As foods containing only minimal protein are eaten during the L-dopa reliant periods, the pH in the stomach is likely to be less acid during these times, unless there is any pathology such as a gastric ulcer.

If the effects of L-dopa medication taken throughout the day are increasingly minimised, the nutritional practitioner would be advised to refer the patient for gastro-intestinal assessment. There could be various reasons, perhaps at the duodenal site, for this. A change of medication to dispersable may be indicated, or a change of L-dopa product to one taken with food.

1.3. Food Facts - For Patients Using Pharmaceutical L-dopa (Problems and Solutions)

People need to ingest carbohydrates, essential fats, minerals, vitamins and protein containing essential amino acids (protein) in order to be able to maintain optimal functional health. Those who are reliant upon L-dopa pharmaceutical medication have certain important considerations to take into account when eating these. Recipes which solve the problems presented in this chapter are to be found in *Part 2*.

Protein

PROBLEM
The amino acids found in protein compete with pharmaceutical levodopa for the absorption sites in the proximal small bowel. Those implicated are the "neutral" amino-acids, tyrosine, phenylalanine, valine, leucine, isoleucine, tryptophane, methionine and histidine. They use the same carrier system for absorption through the gut wall into the blood as they do to penetrate the blood brain barrier. *(26,27)*.

SOLUTION
During the period of time that patients need the effects of pharmaceutical L-dopa, they should only eat foods which contain predominantly carbohydrates or fats (please refer to the food lists in *Part 2*).

Should there be a "window," for example at night, when the patient is not taking levodopa, that would be the time to "balance" the day's diet and introduce "complete protein", i.e. one containing all eight of the essential amino acids - for example, a boiled egg, fish, chicken,soya beans or other pulses in combination, (if pulses are not a problem for the digestion.)

There are a host of wholesome and delicious food options for patients. There is a choice of nutritious complex carbohydrates, fruits and vegetables. An imaginative, energy producing and calorifically adequate diet is possible. The "protein window period", whilst the patient is not on the levodopa, will provide the protein necessary for anabolic cellular function. Predigested free-form amino-acids can also be supplemented during this period to ensure adequate protein intake during the 24-hour period.

Dairy Foods

PROBLEM
Milk, cheese and cream contain a high proportion of protein, competing again for the absorption sites of levodopa.

SOLUTION
Butter may be used but in moderation as it is predominantly fat (saturated).

There are delicious rice milks obtainable as substitutes.

Grains

PROBLEM
Wheat, oats, rye, barley and spelt are grains which contain a sticky substance called *gluten*. This could adhere to the intestinal surface and impede maximum absorption of nutrients. Hypothetically, this could compromise the optimum absorption of levodopa. Other delicious grains such as rice, millet, corn and buckwheat may be used for recipes.

SOLUTION
These grains also contain a fairly high protein fraction. The gluten portion itself is a protein. As such, therefore, these particular grains are not suitable for obtaining the best effects from levodopa.

Soya And Other Pulses

PROBLEM
These do not contain gluten, but have a high proportion of protein, thus not being optimal to levodopa absorption.

SOLUTION

There are other nourishing and delicious grains available, with a more optimal ratio of carbohydrate to protein to avoid absorption problems with levodopa.

Example: brown rice, millet, corn, tapioca, buckwheat. These are available as grains, as flours for baking and cooking and also as pastas.

Soya may be eaten only during the "protein window period" but soya may not be suitable to all. The "protein window period" must be calculated when levodopa has been completely absorbed from the gut and is not necessary for the next few hours, for example at night.

Nuts, Seeds and Pulses

PROBLEM

These contain a high percentage of protein, competing for absorption with levodopa.

SOLUTION

Eat these during the "protein window period", usually at night.

Pulses may prove difficult for the digestion and may not suit everyone. In some cases digestive enzymes could help. It is important to soak pulses over night before boiling 3 times, vigorously for 15 minutes in fresh water each time.

Almonds are alkaline and excellent. Peanuts, cashews and brazil nuts are to be avoided as they contain moulds or toxic substances. Other nuts and seeds are acceptable - sunflower seeds, pumpkin seeds, sesame seeds, almonds, hazelnuts and macadamia nuts.

Seeds are best eaten sprinkled over food in a powdery, crushed-up state for maximum absorption of their nutrients (use a food processor.) These include a good proportion of essential fatty acids as well as zinc, calcium, magnesium and of course, protein. They must always be refrigerated.

Cold pressed oils - first pressing vegetable or seed oils may be used cold as dressings. Unhydrogenated seed margarines may be used but not for cooking.

Stimulants (Alcohol, Tea, Coffee, Chocolate)

PROBLEM

Alcohol is a neurotoxin. This is contra-indicated in patients with Parkinson's Disease. It enters the blood-stream rapidly, causing a sudden release of sugar and thereafter plunges patients into a hypoglycaemic state. This causes mood swings, stress and lack of energy.

SOLUTION

There are excellent substitutes amongst herb drinks, which taste good, look appetising and are refreshing.

PROBLEM

Tea, coffee and chocolate contain stimulants which have the effect of a short-lived spurt of energy and release of sugar into the blood-stream. Soon after, the patient is in a hypoglycaemic state.

This is non-productive as regards stress and energy levels.

SOLUTION

Substitute with refreshing herb teas and "coffee-type" drinks made from other vegetable sources such as chicory or dandelion. Carob, a bean which tastes like chocolate, is a complex carbohydrate and is an excellent alternative.

Yeast

PROBLEM

This contains a very high proportion of protein.

SOLUTION

Bread and confectionary can be made without yeast and there are commercial bouillon cubes which are yeast free.

Balancing Blood Sugar Levels

PROBLEM
As patients with Parkinson's Disease are often lacking in energy and stress can be a problem, it would be advisable to aim for consistency in the control of blood sugar levels.

SOLUTION
Balancing blood sugar levels could be helped by the eating of a regular small snack (for example, every two hours or between meals.) Small portions of complex carbohydrate, ideally with a little raw salad and a drink, should be taken. If indicated, gluten-free Konjac Fibre may be taken (28,29). This is a slow-releasing complex carbohydrate fibre which slows down the absorption of glucose, making for a better sustained energy. The effects of this fibre on L-dopa absorption should be assessed individually as the protein portion, although small, may "compete" for the absorption sites of L-dopa and undermine motor control.

If food is unavailable at "snack time", a drink such as Utra Fuel by TWIN LAB, the American company, usually available in Health Stores, can be drunk. This provides energy and calories and a clear field for L-dopa absorption. It is a fructose based drink with long chain complex carbohydrate polymers.

It is important that ONE bottle only is SIPPED THROUGHOUT THE DAY rather than large quantities drunk at one time. It should be diluted with 50% still water, not to be too taxing to the system. Ultra Fuel is not intended as a food substitute - but as a useful adjunct to boost energy and calories (400 calories per bottle) and to be used for emergencies when food is not available.

Glucose, available from this drink, is essential for the brain. It is usually possible and advisable for the patient to carry, for example, some rice crackers and an apple on his person, as well as a bottle of diluted Ultra Fuel. This ensures a steady boost to energy. It can be used successfully to take L-dopa medication. It has been shown that glucose loading can enhance the efficacy of L-dopa (30). Diabetics should be professionally guided with carbohydrate/glucose loading.

24

1.4. FOODS COMPATIBLE WITH THE ABSORPTION OF LEVODOPA (31,32)

Grains
- Millet
- Rice (Brown and White)
- Tapioca
- Corn (Maize)
- Buckwheat
- Quinoa

Vegetables
- Most, including potatoes, sweet potatoes, turnip, swede, cabbage, cauliflower, carrots, broccoli, courgettes, onions, plantains, yams, pumpkins, squashes (those from the hot countries).
- *But excluding*: Pulses, fresh peas, spinach, asparagus, nuts, seeds or sprouts, e.g. alfalfa, as these contain too high a level of protein.

Oils
- Cold pressed olive oil. This monounsaturated oil must be kept refridgerated and may be used for cooking.
- Cold pressed sunflower, corn, sesame, soy oils. These polynsaturated oils must be kept refridgerated and used for salad dressings. They must never be used for cooking as they produce free radicals which are unhealthy.
- Although whole seeds contain a high proportion of protein, their oils do not.

Herb Teas
- Peppermint (soothing)
- Camomile (soothing)
- Lemon Verbena
- Nettle
- Rooibosch (similar taste to conventional tea)
- Meadow Sweet

Coffee Substitutes

- Chicory (check no wheat added)
- Dandelion (check no wheat added)

Water

Bottled mineral or purified water, preferably "still." Check the water purification system for adequate removal of heavy metals.

Spreads

- Margarine (Non hydrogenated and not containing wheat or dairy products)
- Butter (unsalted)
- Olive spread, e.g. Olive Chalice
- Fruit spreads, e.g. Meridian or other makes sweetened with fruit juice and do not contain refined sugar   (continued overpage)
- Home made aubergine, courgette and onion blended spreads
- Other home-made vegetable spreads, mashed banana or other sliced fruits.

Breads, Biscuits and Cakes

- Gluten free bread, e.g. Sunnyvale Mixed Grain Sourdough Bread, EnerG Brown Rice Bread or home made gluten-free bread and biscuits
- Kallo Rice Crackers or other makes not containing wheat or other high protein content such as soya , nuts and dairy
- Rice Crackers or others not containing wheat or other high protein proportion such as soya, nuts and dairy
- Recipes in this book
- Flours for cooking and baking - rice flour, maize flour, millet flour, buckwheat flour, tapioca flour, potato flour and polenta (a maize product)

Fruit

- All fresh fruits, unless there is a contraindication, e.g. citrus if there is an associated problem
- Tinned fruit sweetened with fruit juice (no added sugar)

- Dried fruit, preferably without artificial colours or preservatives, in moderation, as these have a high sugar content
- Prunes and figs are helpful for intestinal transit

Fruit Juices

- Sugar free (natural). These should always be diluted with 50% still water as the amount of natural sugar is rather high in packeted fruit juices. Concentrates in bottles should also be diluted with still mineral water.

Milk Substitutes

- Rice milk (e.g. Rice Dream)

Social Drinks

May be presented in the same manner as alcoholic drinks, in wine or champagne glasses.

- Sao Rico (contains guarana, a stimulant, so use in moderation mainly as a wine substitute)
- Elderflower
- Ame (white, red or rose)
- High Calorie Energy Drink - Ultra Fuel by Twin Lab, diluted.

Vegetable Stock Cubes Or Powders (Bouillon Cubes)

- Vegetable stock cubes not containing wheat, peanuts or yeast or freshly cooked stock.

1.5. High Proportion Protein Foods for the "Protein Window Period" only

(The duration of the window varies individually dependent on the transit time of the protein ingested)

Proteins Containing Essential Amino Acids:

- Sea Fish (not farmed)
- Eggs (boiled or poached for the optimal effect of lecithin)
- Chicken breasts
- Turkey breasts
- Dairy Products (unless contraindicated)
- Almonds
- Seeds (crushed to powder in a blender or Magimix)
- Sprouts
- Soya (if easily digested)
- Pulses (if easily digested)
- Asparagus
- Spinach (raw only)
- Breads (gluten free)
- Yeast containing foods, e.g. bouillon cubes or Marmite

CAUTION 1: The evening meal during the "protein window period" should be of a "comfortable" size. It should include concentrated protein as above, with vegetables and perhaps fruit. However, there is the temptation to make up for lost time and over-eat. Ensuing digestive discomfort could possibly impede sleep. Also, the transit time of the protein could be delayed. This could theoretically impede the achievement of a "clear field" in the proximal small bowel before the recommencement of levodopa medication. Do not load the meal with heavy carbohydrates at night - green and yellow vegetables with the protein are more suitable.

CAUTION 2: Gluten-containing foods, even during the protein period, should be avoided as gluten could adhere to the gut lining and perhaps impede a clear field at the absorption site for levodopa. Foods containing gluten are: wheat, rye, oats, barley, spelt.

1.6. CONSTIPATION

(The next Chapter describes a routine for alleviating constipation)

This condition is often prevalent in sufferers with Parkinson's Disease. It could be due to different causes such as medication, the illness itself, poor diet, lack of adequate amounts of fibre, insufficient fluids or lack of exercise. Unremitting constipation with pain could possibly often indicate *bowel obstruction* and is an urgent matter for the medical practitioner to assess.

Constipation may perhaps be alleviated by:

- **Fluids**: Sufficient fluids - 2 cups of liquid, preferably at room temperature with each meal. *(33)*. *Also, fluids taken in between meals.*

- **Fibre**: Psyllium Husks in capsule or powder form (capsules are easier because of taste) taken with 2 glasses of liquid (capsules can be more easily swallowed with a little apple sauce in addition to liquid.) However, powder is available to those with swallowing difficulties. *include* stewed Prunes and/or Figs can be included in suitable quantities.

- **Insoluble Fibre:** At each meal there should be sufficient complex carbohydrate containing insoluble fibre. Raw salads, if coped with, are helpful especially when accompanying starchy meals (salads could be finely processed or liquidised if chewing is a problem). Laxative reactions appear to predominate with insoluble fibres. Example: Rice bran has a greater laxative effect than guar. *(34)*.

- **Fresh Fruit:** Fresh fruit is also helpful. Pectin on its own, as a supplement, is not particularly recommended as it slows gastric emptying time. *(35)*. It is more suited to the binding of loose stools.

- **Regular Exercise And Massage:** Regular exercise and massage appropriate to the patient is essential. Specific Isometric Exercises to tone the muscles of the abdominal wall should form part of the programme. Self massage around the large bowel could be useful. The choice of exercise specific to each individual would best be recommended by a physiotherapist.

- **Abdominal Breathing:** Abdominal breathing as a technique is invaluable and can be taught by a physiotherapist.

- **On Visiting the Toilet:** Patients should be encouraged to develop a feeling for reflex bowel movement.

  Twenty minutes after a meal, they should routinely visit the toilet, taking with them a book or some other means of relaxation. Abdominal breathing could form part of this routine. They should not attempt to force a motion, which could lead to prolapsed haemorroids. If a bowel movement is forthcoming, all well and good. If not, after ten minutes the effort should be abandoned until after the next meal or whenever the urge spontaneously arises.

  Anxiety in Parkinson's patients can often exacerbate tremor. Patients should therefore be aware that it is not crucial to have their bowel movements absolutely regularly at the beginning of this regime. Spontaneous peristalsis could very well eventually be induced as a result of this training period, supported by the appropriate fibre and fluid intake. (Wheat bran should not be included among the fibres.) The amount of psyllium husks, prunes and fluids needs to be adjusted perhaps several times until the individual requirement of patients is calculated.

- **Enemas and Suppositories:** If indicated, the patient could be helped on occasion with an enema or the use of glycerine suppositories. Consultation with a specialist in the field of colonic irrigation ("wash-out" therapy) would be helpful.

1.7. A PRACTICAL METHOD FOR ALLEVIATING CONSTIPATION

The choice of method by the patient can only be based on personal experience. However, the Authors have had excellent results with Parkinson's patients using the following method. The next chapter presents fibre containing foods which are helpful in the general diet for alleviating constipation.

Method - using psyllium husks, prunes and extra fluids

10 MINUTES BEFORE BREAKFAST
6 to 8 prunes or 3 figs (as a starting portion) simmered in a little water, pureed if necessary for swallowing. The amount of fruit should be adjusted according to the needs of the individual. Patients should be prepared for trial and error.

BREAKFAST
During your usual breakfast take Psyllium Husks, capsules or powder, as directed. Swallow capsules with a little apple sauce if necessary, as well as liquid for easier swallowing.

2 cups of liquid must accompany them, and can form part of the meal. This can include, for instance, the rice milk in cereal.

N.B.   Keep Psyllium Husks in the fridge.

MID-MORNING
Herb tea or diluted fruit juice and a rice cracker with a little salad.

LUNCH
During the usual lunch take 4 Psyllium Husks or equivalent powder, ensuring that at least 2 glasses of liquid are imbibed during the meal. The amount of 4 Psyllium Husks is merely a suggested recommendation as a starter dose. The patient must be prepared for trial and error in establishing the optimum amount for easy bowel function. The meal should include raw

salad which contains celery, cabbage and carrot. This can be processed finely or even liquidised for swallowing difficulties.

MID-AFTERNOON
Herb Tea or diluted fruit juice plus rice cracker with small salad

DINNER
During the usual dinner take Psyllium Husks with 2 cups fluid at the meal - or as directed.

Alternative times for taking psyllium husks
Should patients find that taking Psyllium Husks is too filling at meal times, they can be taken 3 times daily between meals. However, it is essential that 2 full glasses of water, or fruit juice (diluted) or other liquid be taken at that time. A good time would be with the mid-morning and mid-afternoon snack. Again it should be noted that the amount of Psyllium Husks and the amount of times they are taken daily, are subject to trial and error.

If psyllium husks are used away from main mealtimes, it is essential that at least 2 cups of liquid are still drunk during those main meals and not only when psyllium husks are taken. Constipation requires an optimal amount of fluid, which means at least 10 cups of liquid daily.

Beverage
The following juice could be beneficial drunk hot during the day or before retiring. *It should, however, not form part of a diabetic diet.*

Fig, Prune and Raisin tea - drink warm *(37)*

INGREDIENTS:
- 10-12 figs cut up
- 10-12 prunes cut up
- 2 tablespoons raisins
- 2 pts still mineral water

METHOD

Cover the pot containing the above and simmer gently for 30 minutes. Lemon juice may be added to flavour (if there is no contraindication to citrus.) Strain and keep in the refridgerator. Heat as required.

Toilet Habit

The toilet should be visited 20 minutes after each meal to establish habit reflex. (*36*). There is no need for worry if there is not a resultant bowel movement. One should relax and read a book for 5-10 minutes - no straining or pushing. The toilet should be vacated if there is no subsequent bowel movement. Patients should be aware that it is not crucial to have their bowel movement regularly in the beginning. This is a training period and it is hoped that spontaneous peristalsis will eventually be induced. Should the patient experience continuing constipation and pain, the physician must be contacted immediately to ensure that there is no bowel obstruction.

Enema

An enema may be used under professional supervision only. A professional in colonic irrigation could be helpful. Glycerine suppositories may occasionally be used under supervision.

Osteopathy and Chiropractics:

An assessment by these professionals could prove beneficial. Should the patient require any manipulation, it should be stated that soft tissue work must precede treatment. A request should be made for manipulation to be as gentle as possible.

Exercise and Physiotherapy

Regular exercise appropriate to the patient is essential. A physiotherapist is best consulted about the patient's movement potential. If possible a regular walk in the fresh air is both enjoyable and beneficial.

1.8. FIBRE-CONTAINING FOODS (38)

Bran (wheat or rice) is the most concentrated fibre. It is therefore advisable
to add cooked brown rice to salads and even serve a small portion when
potatoes are eaten. However, in the Optimum Parkinson's Diet, wheat
contains gluten and is therefore excluded. Whole-grain cereals have more
fiber than refined types. Fruit is not exactly a high-fiber food: dark leafy
greens, although containing vitamins and minerals, have little fiber.
However, the quantity of fiber in a food product appears to be less
important than the frequency of consumption.

1. Highest amount of fiber:
    *   Whole grain cereals (corn, wheat, barley, rice, oats, buckwheat,
        millet, rye)
2. A little less fiber:
    *   Legumes (lentils, beans, peas)
    *   Nuts, Seeds
    *   Dried fruits (prunes and figs are popular because a small amount of
        the fruit contains a lot of fiber.)
3. Even less fiber:
    *   Root vegetables (parsnips, potatoes, beets, carrots, turnips)
4. Still less fiber:
    *   Fruits
    *   Leafy vegetables (cabbage, celery, lettuce)
5. No fiber:
    *   Chicken, Meat, Fish, Eggs
    *   Milk and milk products (buttermilk, cheese, yoghurt)
    *   Refined grains, confectionary

It is beneficial to add foods such as celery, lettuce, carrots, radishes and
cabbage to the diet. These readily absorb moisture. There are also foods
which can have a slight laxative effect - raw figs, strawberries, prunes, raw
spinach, water melon, garlic, dandelion leaf tea (without wheat added).
Prunes seem to be especially helpful.

*Melons and prunes should always be eaten away from other foods and
from each other (e.g. 20 minutes before a meal or in between meals.) This
is because they have a very fast transit time through the stomach and if
impeded by other foods, would ferment and cause flatulence.

1.9. STRESS AND DEPRESSION

Depression often appears to afflict the Parkinson's patient. Apart from pathophysiological causes, it would be unnatural if people with the illness were not affected by their symptoms. However, depression may sometimes be exacerbated as a side effect of certain drugs taken. Psychological support must be sought by patient and family or carer.

Many people with Parkinson's disease do find that their symptoms of motor disturbance are exacerbated by stress. Gastrointestinal problems, pH levels and glycaemic controls, amongst other physiological functions, may be influenced by stress. Therefore, if stress control, relaxation and coordination of mind and body are problems, it would be wise to seek help provided by the following:

1. Consultations with a Psychologist, Psychiatrist or Sexual Therapist

2. Autogenic training

3. Biofeedback techniques

4. Meditation

5. Consultations with an Occupational Therapist who can advise on movement related problems

6. Consultations with a Speech Therapist, who could advise on speech techniques and muscular exercises for the facial muscles, including those pertaining to chewing.

7. Exercise, walking, singing and talking to rythmic music

8. Colour, Sound and Music Therapy

9. Specialised exercise suitable to the person's general condition (advised by a Physiotherapist or Exercise Trainer)

10. Consultation with shops for disability aids such as chairs (which are easier to rise from) and blocks to put under the top of the bed (to raise it slightly in case regurgitation is a problem)

11. Consultations with a Dentist and a Dental Hygienist to ascertain whether dentures are properly fitting and to check regularly whether teeth and gums are in good condition. (See the section on anaesthesia in case dental work would benefit from this or sedation)

12. Consultation with shops where specialised cutlery and crockery may be bought to accommodate the special needs of the Parkinson's patient. Cutlery has specially designed handles and plates have raised sides to prevent spillage.

13. If it is difficult to eat or drink because of extreme motor disturbance consideration should be given to the use of naso-gastric feeding or feeding directly into the stomach until physical control is restabilised. This would greatly alleviate stress to the patient.

14. Intravenous infusion (administered very slowly) of vitamins and minerals could be administered, if indicated.

15. Avoid stress in the kitchen through having liquids prepared in thermos flasks. Especially easy are those with a pump mechanism. Have a carer who could prepare and process any foods.

16. A microwave oven, whilst not ideally suitable for cooking at all times, might be a great help as it allows economy of movement and avoids risk of burning arms.

17. A supply of straws which will make drinking easier.

18. Having silk sheets and pyjamas facilitates turning in bed.

1.10. Practical Eating Solutions

(Whether taking l-dopa medication or not)

Eating and drinking could become problematic for some people with Parkinsons disease due either to the disease itself or for other reasons. This could manifest itself as the inability of the patients to physically feed themselves, inability to swallow, lack of appetite due to illness or depression, poor coordination of chewing muscles, dental problems, food intolerances, inflammatory bowel conditions or regurgitation - in addition to many other factors.

All these problems should be considered by the appropriate professional such as the dentist, the nutritionist or dietitian, the occupational therapist, the psychotherapist, the physiotherapist or the medical practitioner.

Supplemental fortified feeding, if not possible orally, should be administered by tube and/or intravenous route, so that the patient does not suffer from malnutrition and lack of energy.

In choosing supplemental feeding it is important to select foods with a predominantly carbohydrate content when needing the effects of L-dopa medication. Protein based foods, possibly including a full spectrum of predigested free-form amino acids, should be given when L-dopa medication is stopped at some point during the 24-hour cycle. This timing is so as not to compromise the absorption potential of the pharmaceutical L-dopa in the small bowel.

If the patient is not on L-dopa medication, Protein based supplemental feeds may be taken freely. Specialised feeding may be in the form of elemental sip feeds, naso-gastric tube feeds, direct feeds into the stomach - or intravenous in extreme cases.

If chewing is a problem, food may be ingested as puree or blended in a liquidizer or food processor.

Physical difficulties with manual control can be addressed by the use of specialised adapted utensils. An Occupational Therapist could guide the patient in this respect.

If there are no problems with chewing or swallowing, normal presentation of food can be enjoyed.

Sublingual, Transdermal, Intravenous and Oral Routes

Tablets, Capsules, Liquids, Powders, Oils, Intravenous Infusions

Some nutritional supplements are available in powder or liquid forms and are easiest to swallow. Tablets may be crushed with a pill crusher and capsules may be emptied. Both may be sprinkled into fruit juice, making for easier swallowing.

If taste permits, fruit juice should be diluted with a little water. However, because of the possible bitter taste of the supplements, it may be necessary to drink the juice in its concentrated form.

Should tablets be be taken, swallowing is facilitated by first moisturising the throat through sipping liquid and then swallowing some smooth fruit puree, such as apple sauce, together with the tablet or capsule *(39)* if help is necessary.

A bottle of water, fruit juice or diluted Ultra Fuel should be kept near or on the person for taking medication or supplements during the day.

Sublingual nutrients are also available and are absorbed directly into the blood.

Oils may be rubbed into the skin for absorption transdermally, alleviating the swallowing problem (onto abdomen, groin area - top of inner upper thigh, inside of upper arm).

Intravenous vitamins and minerals - these may be administered (at a slow rate) in specialised hospital conditions if absorption is a problem.

1.11. Nutritional Management of Patients Undergoing Anaesthesia who are Reliant on L-dopa Medication

1. The night before the operative procedure, for the final evening meal, the patient should eat food which does not require long to digest, e.g. fish or egg, vegetable, salad, fruit. (Protein is included if this is the "protein window period".)

2. Try to organise the operation if possible in the early afternoon so that the normal carbohydrate breakfast may be taken 6 hours before the due time of operation, as well as the levodopa medication.

3. Nothing else may be eaten or drunk before the operation, except for the levodopa medication which must be taken on time as usual, but only with a tiny sip of water.

4. Four hours before surgery the patient should sip about one third of a bottle of a clear carbohydrate-loading drink such as UltraFuel, manufactured by TwinLab, and nothing thereafter.

5. Levodopa must continue to be taken at the usual time with only a sip of water, right up until the commencement of anaesthesia.

6. During anaesthesia only drugs which are not anti-dopaminergic should be used. Drugs which interfere with central amine mechanisms such as phenothiazines and metoclopramide should be avoided where possible; otherwise a close watch should be kept for unusual side-effects.

7. Towards the end of anaesthesia, the anaesthetist could infuse Vitamin C and Vitamin B complex which could enhance recovery.

8. Post-operatively levodopa must be continued at the due times with tiny sips of water as soon as fluids and medication can be taken by mouth.

9. Carbohydrate loading drinks such as UltraFuel, are useful post-operatively when the patient is ready to eat and/or drink.

10. If antibiotics are given to the patient, Probiotics containing L-acidophilis and Bifidobacteria *(40)* should be taken. This regime of replenishing the gut flora should continue for an appropriate period.

11. Caution: some antibiotics, e.g. Flagyl, may cause muscle inco-ordination *(41)*.

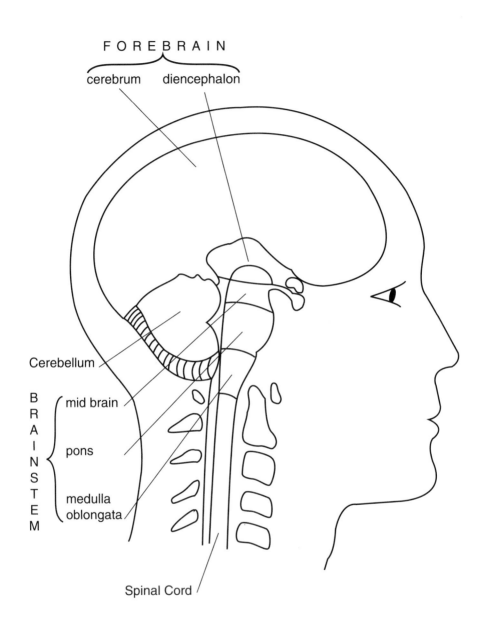

Six divisions of the brain - a simplified sketch.

PART 2

Part 2 is specifically designed for the non-scientific reader. It is user friendly and very easy to follow, meeting both practical and nutritional needs.

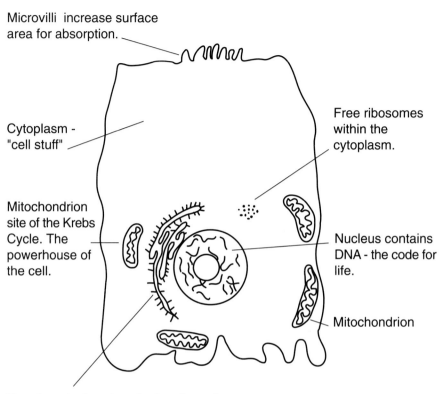

Microvilli increase surface area for absorption.

Cytoplasm - "cell stuff"

Free ribosomes within the cytoplasm.

Mitochondrion site of the Krebs Cycle. The powerhouse of the cell.

Nucleus contains DNA - the code for life.

Mitochondrion

Rough endoplasmic reticulum-bound ribosomes responsible for protein synthesis

A typical animal cell containing a selection of organelles.

2.1. HOW NUTRITION INFLUENCES YOUR BODY

Following are two of many important functions:

How the Body Makes its Own L-dopa and Dopamine

1. Proteins (containing the amino acids which include phenylalanine) are eaten, for example - soya, egg, chicken, milk.

2. In the stomach the protein is processed by hydrochloric acid which uses, amongst other things, zinc and vitamin B6 for its synthesis, and the acid also starts activation of protease enzymes.

3. The processed protein then leaves the stomach and enters the small bowel where it is further digested by protease enzymes. It is then broken down into various amino acids and these are ready to be absorbed through the gut wall into the bloodstream. Absorption occurs at special sites in the gut wall of the small intestine.

4. The blood then carries the amino acids to their destination in the cells of the body.

5. One of the amino acids in certain protein foods is phenylalanine. The blood carries it in a special form to specific neurones (cells) in the brain where dopamine will be made.

6. With the aid of zinc, vitamin B6 (which is broken down to pyridoxine phosphate), vitamin C, glucose and enzymes, the phenylalanine first changes into tyrosine, thereafter into L-dopa and finally into dopamine. Enzymes play a part in all these changes. These enzymes are dependent on minerals such as copper and iron as well as the vitamins C and B6.

It is very interesting to know that tyrosine, which is derived from the original amino acid phenylalanine, can also change into thyroxine which is necessary for thyroid function. It can also become adrenalin and nor-adrenalin (epinephrine and norepinephrine) in the adrenal glands and also goes to form melanin in skin pigmentation.

The Balance Between 3 Neuro-Transmitters; Dopamine, Serotonin And Acetylcholine

It has been suggested that the efficacy of dopamine depends on balanced amounts of itself, serotonin (derived from the amino acid tryptophan in protein) and acetyl choline (which is also synthesized from specific protein foods) *(42)*.

If levels of any of these three elements are disproportionately high or low, Parkinsonian-like symptoms could possibly occur. Nevertheless, even though there may be an optimal intake of these raw materials, other factors may still influence their biosynthesis in people with Parkinson's Disease. Some foods contain free form L-dopa. Soya lecithin granules contain choline and Bananas are a source of tryptophan.

How Cells Make Energy in order to Carry Out their functions

In each cell of the body a process takes place known as the citric acid or Krebs Cycle. The end result of this biochemical process is the production of ATP (Adenosine Tri-Phosphate), which simply means energy for the cell to use.

ATP is produced from Glucose, using B vitamins (1,2,3,5,6), vitamin C, biotin, minerals (magnesium, manganese, iron), co-enzyme Q10, co-enzyme 1 and oxygen.

The Food Programme in this book recommends nutrients to boost the Krebs Cycle and recommends raw materials for the biosynthesis of the neurotransmitters particularly implicated in Parkinson's Disease. However, it must be remembered that there may be other factors present in the Parkinson's Patient which influence the biosynthesis of neurotransmitters. Nonetheless it remains important for the patient to support the body nutritionally as much as possible in order to maintain basic anabolic and catabolic health.

Optimum food sources for glucose are carbohydrates, preferably mainly complex ones such as whole grains and sweet potatoes. Fruit also contains simple carbohydrates. Vitamins and minerals are found in green leafy vegetables and fruit. Oxygenation is enhanced by exercise or special breathing.

With food sources of nutrients being somewhat adulterated in modern times, it could be helpful to take supplements of vitamins, minerals and essential fatty acids under the supervision of a nutritionally trained professional. As carbohydrate loading has been found to enhance dopamine production, your nutritional advisor may see fit to recommend a carbohydrate energy drink such as Ultra Fuel, diluted with water.

CAUTIONARY NOTE: In diabetics the carbohydrate loading needs to be professionally directed at all times.

2.2. SPECIAL PROBLEMS

These topics are to be found in *Part 1*. They are tabulated here in case "non-scientific" readers have omitted to study *Part 1*.

For the following see *Part 1*:

- **CONSTIPATION**   page 29

- **METHODS TO ALLEVIATE CONSTIPATION** page 31

- **FIBRE FOODS**   page 34

- **STRESS AND DEPRESSION**   page 35

- **PRACTICAL EATING**   page 37

2.3. DIET FOR THE PARKINSON'S PATIENT WHO IS NOT ON L-DOPA MEDICATION

Dear Reader,

Your daily diet should be varied and nutritious, free from artificial additives when possible. Eat three meals regularly and have a small snack and drink in between. Don't eat refined and processed foods.

Your food each day should include good quality protein, carbohydrates, essential fatty acids and sufficient fluids. These can be found in fish, poultry, eggs, vegetables including green leafy and yellow/orange types, fruit, nuts, seeds and whole grains.

At least 10 cups of fluid should be imbibed daily. Water should be filtered by reverse osmosis method if possible or use still mineral water. Fruit juices should be sugar free and diluted with water. Avoid caffeine, substituting tea, coffee, alcohol and chocolate with herb teas, chicory, dandelion coffee, refreshing herbal drinks such as Ame or Elderflower and Carob in place of chocololate.

Use only butter or cold pressed olive oil for cooking. Unhydrogenated margarine may be used as a spread.

To help with a comfortable bowel movement, make sure to eat a large helping of stewed prunes daily. Figs are also good for bowel function. If more aid is called for because of intestinal irregularity or constipation, Psyllium Husks taken with a large mug of still water as well as plenty of fluids during the day, are helpful.

Every two hours, have a small snack including a nutritious carbohydrate such as a brown rice cracker with salad or an apple and some almonds. Have something to drink. This mid-meal snack is a boost to your cellular energy and helps to keep your blood sugar even. Drink a diluted bottle (50% water) of the American drink, Ultra Fuel, over the day (found in Chemists, Health or Sports shops). It is great for energy as it is made of long chain glucose polymers.

Use a little fructose or small amount of honey instead of sugar. Try to cut down on sweets and cakes, eating these only on special occasions. There are some excellent recipes for healthy biscuits and cake in the recipe section of this book.

Wheat and cow's dairy foods are best eaten at three day intervals each week. Gluten in wheat may adhere to the intestinal wall, possibly impeding absorption. It is also a very common allergen. Cow's dairy products could also be mucus forming or allergenic in some people. Butter seems to be better tolerated, however. If there is clinical or biochemical evidence demonstrating any food intolerance, the offending food should be eliminated and only reintroduced under supervision of your healthcare professional. Instead, enjoy corn, rice, buckwheat, rye breads and biscuits of those grains. Rice and soya based milks can be used and goat's cheese is a delicious change. Corn and rice cereals are good. Always eat brown rice and whole unrefined grains.

Use the recipes in this book. (You may substitute egg for lecithin as this is for people who cannot eat eggs.)

Enjoy your meals. Bon appetit!

Lucille Leader and Dr Geoffrey Leader

2.4. How to Use and Understand the Diet for Users of L-dopa

Dear Reader,

The success of this dietary programme lies in your understanding of what to choose to eat, and when. *This is really easy, and offers you food which is delicious, simple to prepare and good for family and friends. It gives both energy and good nutrition.*

The important point to remember is that concentrated proteins (meat, fish, chicken, eggs, dairy foods (not butter)) coconut, pulses (for example, chick peas, green peas, lentils, dried beans), spinach and gluten grains (wheat, rye, oats, barley, sago, soya, couscous, bulgar, spelt) interfere with the optimum absorption of medication containing levodopa.

If your L-dopa drug programme is only stopped at night, after your last drug has been taken, wait 1 hour and thereafter enjoy a meal containing concentrated protein. Your L-dopa drug may have already been absorbed after 1 hour and the proteins that you eat should not upset its absorption as such. Note that during a 24-hour cycle you will have eaten a normal balanced diet containing carbohydrates and fats mainly for energy and general nutrition during the day, adding proteins at night, ensuring the essential amino acids needed.

If you need another boost of L-dopa before going to sleep, only if possible wait 2 hours after the protein meal and before taking it. This is in case your protein meal has not yet passed the special absorption site in your small bowel.

However, experience will be your teacher! If you need the help of your L-dopa medication sooner than 2 hours, take it and see whether your tremor/dyskinesia is affected. If there is exacerbation of symptoms, you will know that the protein you ate did require longer to pass by the special absorption sites.

Example

If you are off levodopa from 6 p.m. to 8 a.m., your eating choices could be as follows:

Breakfast: Carbohydrates and fats, e.g. cereals, rice milk, corn toast and a scraping of butter and fruit spread, herb tea, fruit

Tea break: Carbohydrates and fats, e.g. rice crackers or corn/rice toast with butter, vegetable pate or avocado and tomato, herb tea or fresh vegetable soup, fruit juice or dilute Ultra Fuel

Lunch: Carbohydrates and fats, e.g. soups, jacket potato and scraping of butter, potato latkes or rosti, rice pasta and tomato based sauce, salad with olive oil and lemon dressing, fruit, juice or still mineral water, etc.

High Tea: Carbohydrates and fats, e.g. vegeburger or corn pasta and salad with dressing, fruit, dilute Ultra Fuel, herb teas or soup

Dinner: (at least 1 hour after last L-dopa tablet) Proteins should be added to your usual meal of carbohydrates and fats, e.g. chicken, fish, vegetable, salad, fruit, rice pudding, carob cake, almonds, fruit juice, still mineral water, herb teas

Remember to eat a snack between meals as illustrated above. This snack is for energy and the fluids drunk during the day will help the problem of constipation.

Choices and Preparation

Preparation Of Carbohydrates

Carbohydrates, particularly complex carbohydrates, provide energy, vitamins and minerals. When choosing carbohydrates, preferably use unrefined foods such as brown rice instead of white. Leave on the potato jackets (skins) of sweet and ordinary potatoes, and eat them. Carbohydrates, particularly complex carbohydrates, provide energy, vitamins and minerals. If there is a problem, leave off the skins. If swallowing is difficult, blend the foods in a blender or food processor.

Eat plenty of yellow vegetables, e.g. squashes, plantains, pumpkins and carrots as well as green vegetables. Steam vegetables with the lid of the pot tightly closed, as the preferred cooking technique. Plantains should be boiled in a little water in a covered pot.

Nuts and seeds, however, although concentrated carbohydrate, also contain a high proportion of protein. Only take these during the "protein period." Their oils contain virtually no protein.

Sweeteners: use Manuka honey (preferably), molasses or fructose should be used instead of conventional sugars. Refined sugars are stimulants which are contraindicated.

Preparation Of Fats

Butter may be used at any time, in moderation. Although butter comes from a dairy product which contains concentrated protein, by the end of its manufacture it contains only saturated fat. Butter may be heated or used cold.

Margarine may only be used if unhydrogenated as well as polyunsaturated. Hydrogenated, polyunsaturated margarines are not healthy *(43)*. Do not heat or cook with margarine, as this produces free radicals which are contraindicated and extremely unhealthy.

The only oil used for cooking should be cold-pressed olive oil. This is a monounsaturated oil which is more stable than the polyunsaturated product. It can be used for salad dressings too.

Oils for salad dressings may be cold-pressed polyunsaturated oils such as sunflower, safflower and corn oils, but these should never be heated because of their production of free radicals.

It is most important to keep any oil in the refrigerator. This is because oils rapidly become rancid. Nuts and seeds also contain polyunsaturated oils and should be kept in the refrigerator.

Protein Foods

Enjoy these when pharmaceutical L-dopa is not relied upon for its effects, and the last dose has been completely absorbed.

- Boiled or poached eggs - these are best as lecithin, contained therein for emulsifying cholesterol, is still intact.
- Sea fish - not "farmed " or river fish as they may contain undesirable chemicals.
- Skinless white of chicken - the brown contains a high proportion of saturated fats. Skinless white or brown of turkey.
- Almonds or other nuts - no cashews, peanuts or brazil nuts as these may contain moulds or toxins.
- Seeds - (crushed for absorption) can be eaten to provide essential amino acids.
- Soya - if digestion permits. Follow directions for pre-soaking before cooking (see page 22)
- Pulses - if digestion permits. Follow directions for pre-soaking before cooking (see page 22.)

Remember to give these foods at least 2 hours' clearance time, if possible, before recommencing medication containing levodopa. They must pass beyond the area in the proximal small bowel where they compete for absorption sites with the levodopa.

If you cannot wait 2 hours, you will have to see what suits you best.

Tea, Coffee, Chocolate, Alcohol
Use herb teas and coffee alternatives such as chicory and carob (an alternative to chocolate.) These are delicious, refreshing and do not zap energy, upsetting blood sugar levels, as do stimulant drinks.

Additives And Additions
Do not buy food containing preservatives, chemical additives or sugars other than honey or fructose. Limit salt (sodium chloride) or, better still, leave it out relying on herbs for flavour and natural sodium found in vegetables. Sodium in the best bioavailable form can always be supplemented if indicated (44).

Water
Only use still mineral water or filtered waters in order to avoid heavy metals and bacteria. Sparkling water is not ideal as it causes an acid condition in the gut and could also precipitate bloating.

Social Outings

The foods available to you are a pleasure to eat as well as providing health-giving nutrients. Always take a purse or bag with you when you go out, containing some herb tea bags and a little bottle of still mineral water. The water could also be mixed with some Ultra Fuel for extra energy.

If you go out for dinner or on another social occasion to friends, let them know if you are in the levodopa period and ask for vegetables and fruit - e.g. jacket potatoes and butter, or rice, vegetable, salad and fruit. Remember, however, that soya and other pulses do have a high protein content. This should present no problems at all to your host. Many people are vegetarians or vegans today.

Restaurants are no problem - there are always plenty of choices.

Home Dinner Parties

Whatever the time of day, your food choice is attractive and nutritious enough to be enjoyed alike by friends and family.

Be adventurous with new recipes!

Fill your wine glasses with chilled herb drinks or fruit juices. Present these in attractive carafes.

Enjoy your food! Bon appetit!

Lucille Leader and Dr. Geoffrey Leader

2.5. LIST OF *'GOOD'* FOOD TYPES

(Whether using L-dopa medication or not)

Carbohydrates

- Buckwheat (flour and grains and pasta)
- Brown rice (flour and grains)
- Millet (flour and grains)
- Tapioca (flour and grains)
- Maize (flour and grains)
- Plantains
- Potatoes (sweet and ordinary)
- Potato flour
- Pumpkin
- Squashes
- Gluten-free cereals
- Polenta
- Rice and Maize Pastas (corn)
- Popcorn
- Potato crisps (sparingly as they contain heated oils)
- Rice crackers and other gluten-free biscuits
- Corn crackers
- Carob
- Fruit
- Vegetable sauces
- Yams

Fats

- Cold-pressed olive oil is a monounsaturated fat. It can be heated or used as a dressing.
- It may be used at all times and stored in a refridgerator.
- Butter contains mainly saturated fat and may be used sparingly at all times.
- Cold-pressed sunflower, sesame and safflower oils are polyunsaturated fats which must be stored in a refridgerator. They may not be heated.
- Coconut milk contains saturated fat and protein but no cholesterol, and can be used moderately during the "protein window period" only.

Proteins

Note: List Of healthy proteins to be used during the "Protein Window Period" and for others not on L-dopa Medication

- Boiled or poached eggs (preferably), although eggs may be cooked or used in other ways
- White of chicken. Brown and white of turkey (skinless) Avoid red meat
- Sea fish
- Smoked fish (eat only occasionally as smoked foods can be carcinogenic.)
- Soya beans - providing digestion is not a problem. If not ready-made, note directions prior to cooking (see page 22)
- Lentils and other pulses - providing digestion is not a problem. If not ready-made, note directions for soaking prior to cooking (see page 22.)

2.6. ALTERNATIVE FOODS TO USE WHEN NEEDING THE EFFECTS OF L-DOPA

(Giving List of Unsuitable Foods with Good Substitutes)

Note: Brand names of products recommended are only a guide. Equally appropriate makes surely exist in different areas. The important issue is to check the contents of the products on offer.

WRONG FOODS	GOOD SUBSTITUTE FOODS
Gluten containing foods:	
Wheat, rye, oats, barley, sago, couscous, spelt, bulgar, gram flour (chickpeas)	Rice, millet, tapioca, maize, buckwheat (as flours, flakes or crumbs, mixed into different foods for baking, batter or for thickening), potato flour, polenta
Breads, biscuits, rolls (unless gluten free)	Those marked "gluten free" and not containing other high protein content foods, example eggs or soya. Use a combination of rice, millet and buckwheat flours to make home-made breads, biscuits and cakes. Home made or bought polenta is corn based.
Cakes and pancakes containing gluten	Substitute a mixture of rice, millet, buckwheat and/or maize flours to make cakes. Use rice flour in pancakes.
Cereals (unless gluten free), Gluten free muesli containing high protein grains or flakes	Cornflakes (Evernat Organic sweetened with apple juice, no added wheat) Rice Krispies (Kallo without additions of other substances)
Baking powders (unless gluten free)	Gluten free baking powders at health shops and chemists.
Crumbles	Use butter blended with rice flour to make crumbs. Sprinkle them over fruit, vegetables, fish or chicken

Condiments - chutneys, mustards, ketchups, soya sauce, curry powders	Gluten free varieties: tomato sauce (home-made) or tomato ketchup (Life & Heinz), fruity brown sauce (Life), curry powder without wheat or gluten, sieved tomatoes, tomato puree, chopped tomatoes
Vinegars, - spirit, wine, malt, etc.	Apple cider vinegar, Lemon juice, Fresh limes
Gravy powders, stock cubes	Those marked gluten free if ready made OR make home-made stock. Thicken gravies with rice flour or maize flour which is used in exactly the same way as wheat flour
Yeast containing foods: Baker's yeast, Marmite, some bouillon cubes	Low yeast breads, example sour dough, and bouillon cubes which are yeast free
Pastas (wheat)	Rice pasta (Orgran), rice vermicelli (Chinese rice noodles), corn pasta, buckwheat pasta
Sauce mixes and ready-made soups (unless gluten free)	Home-made sauces from fresh ingredients and thickened with rice flour

Concentrated proteins:	
milk of animals, coconut milk, seed milk	Rice milk (Rice Dream)
Red meat, chicken, turkey and fish	Free range or organic chicken and turkey Sea fish only (not framed)
Smoked foods	Limit smoked foods as these could be carcinogenic
Instant Puddings	Home-made tapioca pudding, home-made rice pudding, home-made rice noodle pudding or blended fruits
Alcoholic drinks	Ame, Elderflower, Aqua Libra and other non-sugar containing herb drinks (no artificial sweeteners); fruit juices diluted with a third still water

Tea	Herb teas, particularly camomile, peppermint and meadowsweet
Coffee	Chicory (Prewetts)
Chocolate	Carob
Spreads	Home-made vegetable spreads; fruit spreads (Meridian); Olive Spread. Butter may be used moderately as it contains only saturated fat
Cocktail or TV snacks	Corn crackers, tacos (wheat free); popcorn (if home made use olive oil); potato crisps (as they contain vegetable oil of unknown origin, use sparingly); rice crackers with vegetable pate or fruit spread; butter may be used; crudites with avocado pear dip; vegeburgers (made with rice flour); potato latkes; dips, pates, e.g. aubergine, onion, courgettes and peppers sauteed together and used as a dip.
Vegetable oils	Use only cold pressed olive oil or a little butter for cooking (polyunsaturated oils, when heated, produce a greater cascade of free radical activity.) Use cold pressed polyunsaturated oils cold, for salad dressings only. Example, corn oil, safflower oil, sunflower oil, marked 'cold-pressed' on the bottle. Keep these refrigerated.
Margarine	Only non-hydrogenated margarines (*not for cooking*) Butter is sparingly allowed (*as a spread and for cooking*)

2.7. ESSENTIAL PRACTICAL ADVICE

By following these helpful tips, your cooking should be safe and enjoyable!

1. Obtain help to chop up food ready for cooking.

2. Keep food in special food or freezer bags.

3. Try to obtain help in preparing a week's amount of food. Keep it in your freezer or fridge. Warm up as needed..

4. If you do not have the help of family or friends to prepare foods routinely for you, do speak to your local social services department, social worker, general practitioner or Parkinsons support group. Day Care Centres might also be able to advise you and provide meals. In most areas there are "Meals on Wheels" services, a service delivering food to the home. You would need to advise them of your "special needs diet".

5. Consider the relative safety, when you are on your own, of cooking in an approved stainless steel microwave oven. This requires relatively little physical effort to programme when coordination is a problem. Remember to use specialised microwave-safe dishes, as indicated by the manufacturer.

6. Always use stainless steel or glass cookware. Aluminium is contra-indicated for people with Parkinson's Disease.

7. Obtain specially designed utensils which help to compensate for lack of muscular coordination. An occupational therapist could guide you in this respect.

8. Make sure that you have smoke alarms in strategic and convenient positions in your home.

9. Make sure that you have a small and a large fire blanket in an easily accessible place in the kitchen. In case of fire simply throw a blanket over the flames and do not lift it up until the fire is completely extinguished. Turn off cooker. Blankets could be more practical than a fire extinguisher as they require less physical control in their

administration. However, a fire extinguisher should also form part of kitchen safety. This must be routinely checked for safe functioning.

10. Do keep some sort of treatment for cuts or burns in the kitchen cupboard, including some antiseptic fluid, plasters and simple bandages.

11. Cupboards and drawers should be at a comfortable height.

12. Keep a telephone in the kitchen. Pre-set numbers, for example for emergency services, making for easy dialling, would be helpful.

13. Keep a small bell in your pocket in order to be able to call for help if needed. In some instances it might be helpful to wear an alarm call button on your person. There are specialist firms who provide this service.

14. Keep insulated thermos jugs, with a pump mechanism if possible, filled with hot water, soup or tea. Have your helper fill these for you each day.

15. Use flexible plastic straws which make for easier drinking, and light-weight cups with a handle suited to easy grasp.

16. Rubber mats placed under utensils and plates keeps them from sliding.

17. Use of a pill-box with an alarm is very helpful when times of medication are crucial.

2.8. RECIPES FOR GENERAL USE INCLUDING THE L-DOPA PERIOD

Note: If not using L-dopa, you can substitute egg for lecithin whenever listed

Soups

IMPORTANT NOTE: If using a food processor or chopping food is a problem, just cook the vegetables whole and eat the soup with them in this form.

Satisfying Winter Soup
serves 4

- 3 potatoes, cut into medium-size chunks
- 1 medium onion
- Pumpkin pieces (peeled), quantity as desired
- 1 gluten-free bouillon cube
- 1 celery stick, cut in large pieces

- 1 carrot
- 1 bunch parsley
- 1 courgette
- 2 tomatoes, chopped
- 1 leek (cut in two)
- 1 litre of water

1. Boil all the ingredients in 1 litre of purified or still mineral water. Cover and simmer on medium heat.
2. As soon as vegetables are soft, remove from water and liquidize in a food processor or mash with potato masher.
3. Return blended mixture and purified or still mineral water to pan, heat and serve.

Leek And Tomato Soup
serves 4

- 1 Tbsp. olive oil (cold-pressed)
- 1 clove garlic, crushed
- 1 large onion
- 1 leek, cut in two
- 6 tomatoes
- 1 tsp. fresh thyme
- 1 litre of vegetable stock (made with purified or still mineral water)
- 1 Tbsp. tomato puree
- 1 large potato
- Crushed black pepper (optional)

1. Bring all the ingredients to boil in a soup pot
2. Cover and simmer until vegetables are tender.
3. Blend vegetables in a food processor or mash with a potato masher. Add back to the liquid and serve.

Note: If blending is difficult, eat soup with the vegetables whole.

Gazpacho Soup
serves 4

- 5 large tomatoes, chopped
- 1 clove garlic, crushed
- 1/2 cup celery, diced
- 1 cup cucumber, grated
- 1/2 cup green pepper, diced
- 1/2 cup sweet red pepper, diced
- 1 cup tomato juice
- 1/4 cup fresh parsley, chopped
- 2 Tbsp olive oil (cold-pressed)
- 2 tsp basil, chopped
- Black pepper (optional)

1. Combine all ingredients in a large bowl or food processor. Mix well and chill in refrigerator and serve cold.

Minestrone Vegetable Soup
serves 4

- 1 or 2 chopped onions
- 1 cup chopped tomatoes or
- sieved tomatoes
- 2 carrots, diced
- 3 pints of home-made vegetable stock or 1 bouillon cube (made with purified or still mineral water)
- Black pepper (optional)

- 1/4 of a light cabbage (shredded)
- 1 parsnip (sliced)
- 6 baby potatoes (or larger potatoes cut as desired)
- 3 courgettes (chopped as desired)
- Fresh parsley, as desired

The amount of vegetables is merely a guideline. Any amount of vegetable of any sort combined, makes a delicious soup. The addition of a bouillon cube, without yeast, particularly one with an onion flavour, will improve the flavour.

1. Combine all your ingredients in a large saucepan, with as much purified or still mineral water as you require to cover vegetables.
2. Put the lid on, bring to the boil and thereafter simmer for up to an hour or until the vegetables are soft.

Note: If you find it difficult to chop the vegetables, cook them whole and eat the soup in this way. You can buy many frozen vegetables, already chopped up.

Vichyssoise

serves 4

- 4 potatoes
- 1 large leek
- 1 large onion
- 1 onion soup or other bouillon cube

- 1 pt water (purified or still mineral)
- Black pepper to taste

1. Put all the ingredients into a pot and cook until soft.
2. Blend the vegetables to a smooth liquid in a food processor and then add back to the water.
3. Serve hot or chilled with fresh chopped parsley to decorate.

Note: if chopping is a problem, cook the vegetables whole and eat the soup in this form.

Salads and Salad Dressings

Note: If you are unable to eat citrus fruits, substitute lemon juice with tomato juice for excellent results.

Potato Salad

serves 2

- 4 potatoes (in skins)
- 1 celery stick (chopped)
- 1 apple (chopped)
- 2 spring onions (chopped)
- A sprinkling of chives (chopped)

- Dressing made with 3 Tbsp cold pressed olive oil and 1 Tbsp lemon juice (or tomato juice) crushed garlic and black pepper

Mix the ingredients together in a bowl and toss with the salad dressing.

Pepper And Tomato Salad
Serves 2

- 1 pepper (red, green or yellow)
- 2 tomatoes (finely sliced)

- Dressing made with 3 Tbsp cold pressed olive oil and 1 Tbsp lemon juice (or tomato juice), crushed garlic and black pepper to taste

Salade Paysane
Serves 4

- Green lettuce
- Tomatoes
- Cucumber
- Avocado pear

- Dressing made with 3 Tbsp cold pressed olive oil and 1 Tbsp lemon juice (or tomato juice), crushed garlic and black pepper to taste

1. Combine all salad ingredients in a large bowl.
2. Combine all dressing ingredients into a jar, tighten the lid and shake vigorously till well blended.
3. Pour dressing over salad, toss well and serve.

Carrot Salad
Grate as many carrots as desired and serve either mixed through with soaked sultanas, orange or pineapple juice, or on their own.

Vegetarian Grain Recipes (Gluten Free and Low Protein)

Simple Rice Recipe
Serves 2

- 1 cup white rice
- 2 cups water (purified or still mineral water)
- 1 yeast-free bouillon cube for flavouring (optional)

1. Wash rice 3 times in cold water.
2. Put rice and water together in a pot.
3. Bring to boil.
4. Stir once.
5. Put lid on and simmer on a low heat for 20 minutes.
6. If rice is still moist, leave to simmer a few minutes longer. However, if the rice is still hard, add a little more water and simmer on a low heat for a further few minutes with the lid on until rice is tender.

For Brown Rice:
Use the same recipe as for white rice, but add an extra cup of water.

It will take longer to cook - about 40-50 minutes.

A *delicious variation* when cooking rice is to put some handfuls of sultanas into the water, and a little tomato sauce.

In a separate pan you could saute some chopped up bananas, spring onions and dried ginger flakes in a little olive oil. When these are turning golden, pour them with the oil into the already cooked rice and mix through.

Vegetable Risotto
serves 6

- 8 oz. brown rice
- 1 celery stick, diced
- 1 medium onion, chopped
- 1 courgette, diced
- 8 oz. beansprouts

- 4 oz. sweetcorn kernels
- 8 oz. broccoli florets
- 2 tomatoes, diced
- 1 Tbsp olive oil (cold-pressed)

Note: You can use any vegetable of your choice.

1. Cook rice as package directs.
2. Blanch vegetables for a few seconds in boiling water.
3. Heat olive oil in wok or large pan and stir-fry all vegetables until tender.
4. Add cooked rice to the wok or pan, mix well and heat through. Serve.

Millet Delight
serves 4

- 375g/12 oz millet
- 450ml/ 3/4 pt purified or still mineral water
- 50g/2 oz sultanas or raisins
- 4 tbs oil
- 1 large onion, sliced
- 2 small leeks, sliced

- 1 stick celery, sliced
- 1 clove garlic, crushed
- 2 carrots, diced
- 125g/4 oz mushrooms, sliced
- 2 tbs parsley or chives, finely chopped

1. Wash the millet well in cold running water, drain and put into a pan with the water.
2. Bring to the boil, then cover and simmer until the water is absorbed. Set aside.
3. Heat the oil, fry the onion until soft, stir in all the other vegetables and sultanas, cover, cook for 15 minutes stirring occasionally.
4. Add the cooked millet, cover and cook for 15-20 minutes more. Serve on its own.

Countryside Peppers

serves 6

- 6 medium red/yellow/orange peppers
- 3 cups water (purified or still mineral water)
- 1 cup millet
- 1 1/2 cups onion, chopped
- 1 clove garlic, crushed
- 1/2 cup mushrooms, diced
- 1 Tbsp olive oil (cold-pressed)
- Crushed black pepper (optional)

1. Blanch peppers in boiling water. Allow to cool slightly.
2. Bring water and millet to a boil. Reduce heat. Cover and simmer for 30 minutes.
3. In a pan heat oil and saute garlic, onion and mushrooms. Season to taste.
4. Combine cooked millet, and add to onion mixture.
5. Fill peppers with millet mixture. Bake at 180/350F for 30 minutes, then serve.

Polenta Aux Tomates
serves 6

- 2 pints purified or still mineral water
- 8 oz yellow cornmeal
- 1-2 oz. Butter
- 1 tsp fresh basil
- Sauce
- 1 tsp fennel seed
- 2 Tbsps. olive oil (cold-pressed)
- 1 clove garlic, crushed

- 1 medium onion, chopped
- 1/2 tsp fructose (health food shop)
- 1 lb. chopped tomatoes
- 3 Tbsps. tomato puree
- 1 tsp fresh oregano
- Crushed black pepper (optional)

1. Bring the water to a boil in a large saucepan. Gradually add it to the cornmeal, continually stirring to avoid lumps. Add butter, continuing to cook over a low flame for 20 minutes. The mixture should have a creamy consistency. If not it may be necessary to add more butter/water.
2. Pour into a 13 x 9 inch baking tin, level and set aside to cool.
3. Meanwhile, prepare sauce by heating oil in a saucepan, saute garlic and onion till tender, then add oregano, basil, fennel seeds and black pepper. Stir in chopped tomatoes and puree, add fructose, cover and simmer for 20-30 minutes or until sauce thickens.
4. Slice polenta into squares, cover with sauce and serve.

Note: Polenta may be bought "ready made" at Delicatessen Shops. If using it, re-heat or grill the polenta, make the sauce and cover thin slices of polenta with it.

Potato Delights

Mouth-Watering Potato Latkes
serves 4

- 4 medium potatoes (2 sweet and 2 plain
- 1 dessertspoonful of lecithin granules
- 2 onions
- 2 Tbsps. brown rice flour
- 2 Tbsp. olive oil (cold-pressed)

1. First chop the potatoes and and onions into quarters. Place in a food processor together with the flour, lecithin granules and 2 Tbsp. of olive oil. Chop to a coarse, smooth mixture but do not allow to become a liquid. If watery, add a little more rice flour.
2. Heat a frying pan or griddle with a dash of olive oil, sufficient so that the latkes will not stick to the bottom. Keep heat at medium setting.
3. Drop the mixture by the dessert spoon into pan or onto griddle (mixture should form a mini pattie), cover but keep checking to make sure latkes don't burn or stick. Flip over when lightly browned and cook underside. Total cooking time for each should be about 20 minutes or until the potatoes are cooked through.

Alternative method:

The latkes may be grilled or baked.

Lightly grease an oven dish or baking tin with olive oil. Drop spoonfuls of potato mixture into the dish and pour a little olive oil over each one. Cover with tin foil. Keep under the grill or very hot oven until the potato is cooked through. Take off the tin foil about 10 mins before serving in order to crisp and brown the latkes.

Potato Salad

serves 4

- 4 potatoes with skin

- Dressing of 6 Tbsps olive oil, 2 Tbsps lemon juice or tomato juice, pressed garlic and pepper to taste

1. Cut up potatoes and steam until soft.
2. Prepare dressing and fold in the potatoes.
3. Serve with a salad.

Jacket Potatoes With Butter

serves 4

- Potatoes (preferably sweet or also plain)

- Butter

1. Scrub clean the skins of sweet or ordinary potatoes and prick the potatoes with a fork.
2. Microwave as per instructions. Alternatively oven bake the potatoes, brushed with a little olive oil and wrapped first in greaseproof paper and then in aluminium foil. Make sure that the aluminium foil completely covers the greaseproof paper or it will catch alight in the oven.
3. Bake at 190 degrees C for an hour and a half or until soft.
4. Serve with butter and a salad, or steamed vegetables.

Roast Potatoes

serves 6

- 6 potatoes in jackets, (sweet or usual). *(Pumpkin can also be used)*

- Olive oil

1. Steam potatoes until soft.
2. Coat potatoes with cold-pressed olive oil.
3. Roast in the oven at 190C in an open dish. Turn potatoes intermittently and eat when crisp.

Mediterranean Potatoes (Gluten-Free)

- 4 potatoes
- 1 Tbsp olive oil
- 2 oz/50g unsalted butter
- 1 clove garlic, crushed
- 1 medium onion
- Freshly ground black pepper

- 1 green pepper, seeded and sliced
- 1 tsp mixed herbs
- 14oz/400g tin tomatoes

1. Scrub potatoes and cut into halves or quarters. Steam in a covered dish till the potatoes are done. Put aside.
2. Meanwhile, heat the oil and butter in a frying pan, add garlic, onion and pepper and cook for 5 minutes.
3. Add tomatoes and their juice, breaking up the tomatoes, then add the herbs and seasoning. Cook for 10 minutes.
4. Pour the sauce over the potatoes and serve hot.

Alternatively:

Put all your ingredients , uncooked, into an oven casserole with a cup of water. Cover with tin foil and cook at 180 C for about a 1 or 2 hours or until cooked.

Cakes Biscuits and Pastry

Gluten Free Fruit-Chip Buiscuits

- 200 grammes butter
- 1 1/2 cups brown sugar OR 3/4 cup fructose (fruit sugar)
- 2 Tbs lecithin granules/egg replacer
- 2 tsp vanilla essence

- 1 3/4 cups rice flour
- 1/4 cup buckwheat flour
- 1/4cup millet flakes
- 1 tsp baking soda - bicarb.
- 1 cup chopped fruit

1. Cream butter, sugar, lecithin, vanilla.
2. Add the dry ingredients and mix thoroughly.
3. Add fruit and mix.
4. Form into cookies and bake on a greased baking tray for about 10 minutes at 190C.

Gluten Free Pastry (45)

- 5 oz brown rice flour
- 3 oz millet or buckwheat flour
- 5 oz butter

- 2 large sheets of grease-proof paper

1. Preheat oven to 190 degrees C/375 degrees F.
2. Combine dry ingredients, mixing in oil with a fork.
3. Add water to mixture to form a dough.
4. This pastry is tricky to roll so you might like to do it between grease-proof paper.
5. Sprinkle the lower piece with rice flour, place dough on it, then lay sheet of grease-proof paper on top and flatten with a rolling pin. When it is rolled remove top piece of paper and carry dough to dish on bottom piece of paper. Invert dish onto it, then turn dish right way up, allowing pastry to fall into it. Push into shape. Alternatively, you can roll it out carefully, using plenty of rice flour. Prick well all over then bake blind* for about 25 mintues until set but not hard.
6. Use with your favourite filling, vegetables in tomato puree with a little fresh garlic and spring onion, or pureed fruit.

Alternatively: process an equal amount of butter and rice flour in a food processor. Roll out as desired. Example: 6 ozs rice flour and 6 ozs butter.

*To bake blind, line the oven dish with pastry, cover with grease-proof paper and weight this down with a small quantify of rice grains to hold the paper down and absorb moisture. This seems to make the pastry more crunchy.

Desserts

Note: See previous section on Breads, Biscuits and Pastry for Gluten-free pastry to make bases for your favourite fruit fillings.

Fabulous Crepes

serves 1

- 2 heaping dessertspoons brown rice flour
- 1 dessertspoonful of lecithin
- 2 dessertspoons rice milk
- granules
- Olive oil (cold-pressed) or butter

1. In a mixing bowl, beat lecithin with milk. Gradually add the beaten ingredients to the rice flour stirring into a slightly thick but creamy consistency.
2. Coat a medium size pan with olive oil or butter and heat keeping flame at medium setting. Pour mixture into pan. As soon as bubbles appear on surface (or check underside to see if set) turn over.
3. Serve rolled with fruit spread filling (Meridian/Whole Earth) or organic honey.

Luxury Lokshen Pudding

serves 6

- 1/2 packet of Chinese rice noodles or egg replacer
- 1 tablespoon of lecithin granules
- 1 jar of fruit spread (Meridien/Whole Earth
- 2 handfuls raisins or sultanas (unsulphured or organic)
- 4 apples, cored, peeled and grated

1. Preheat oven to 100C/200F
2. In a small bowl, soak raisins or sultanas in boiling water to soften.
3. Meanwhile boil noodles as package directs. Drain.
4. In a mixing bowl, mix fruit spread, lecithin, grated apples, raisins and noodles together. Add the drained noodles and mix through.
5. Lightly grease a square baking dish with olive oil and place noodle mixture in the dish.
6. Bake for 35 minutes or until lightly browned.

Apple Crumble
serves 2

- 4 chopped sweet eating apples, steamed with a little water until tender
- Manuka honey or fructose to taste
- Butter to grease dish
- Crumbs made from butter and soft rice flour blended together (sufficient to cover apple puree)
- Cinnamon to taste

1. Grease baking dish with butter.
2. Pour the pureed apple into the dish, mixed with sweetener and cinnamon. Sprinkle with the crumbs and bake for 1/2 hour or until the crumbs are brown, at 200F.

Baked Apples
Allow one apple per person

- Cored sweet cooking apples
- Cinnamon
- Manuka honey
- Soaked sultanas or raisins
- Butter
- Cloves

1. Grease baking dish with butter.
2. Stuff the apples with the sultanas, honey and stick a few cloves round the top of the apple.
3. Cover the dish with foil and bake at the bottom of the oven for approximately 1 hour at 180F or until soft.

Fruit Whirl

serves as required

- Chilled fruit:
- Apple
- Banana

- Mango
- Passion fruit
- or fruits of your choice

No melon or plums, as these ferment when together or with other foods.

Whirl in a blender or food processor and serve in a festive glass decorated with a sprig of mint. If eating during the "protein window period", sprinkle with chopped nuts and seeds (which have been blended in a food processor.) Remember to keep the nuts and seeds in the refridgerator.

2.9. CONCENTRATED PROTEIN RECIPES

(for during the "Protein Window Period" and for All)

Use your favourite recipes for chicken, turkey, fish, eggs, pulses, limited amount of cream and coconut.

Remember NEVER include foods containing gluten such as wheat, rye, oats, barley and spelt and NEVER include proteins which cause you digestive discomfort such as flatulence, bloating, constipation or diarrhoea.

Alcohol is a neurotoxin and is not good for you, nor are refined puddings and confectionery! However, there are many satisfying substitutes such as those given on the following pages.

WARNING: It is important not to over-eat at this meal, particularly if it is at night. Protein requires longer than carbohydrates for complete digestion. Overloaded digestive conditions could be uncomfortable and impede sleep and transit time through the digestive tract.

Main meals

Tomato Chicken
serves 4

- 4 breasts of chicken/turkey or whole chicken
- Heinz tomato sauce
- Onion
- Chicken bouillon cube
- Potato and sweet potato
- Green pepper

- 2 cups purified or still mineral water
- A few basil leaves
- 4-6 dessertspoonsful olive oil
- 2 Apples, quartered (optional)

1. Chop onion, pepper, apples, potato, basil leaves. Put into a cooking pot or baking casserole with the chicken. Sprinkle bouillon cube over ingredients. Cover chicken completely in tomato sauce and olive oil.
2. Only add a little water, because a thick sauce is more delicious.
3. Cook gently on top of the stove for 1 to 2 hours in a covered pot or until the chicken is soft. Check liquid level frequently. Stir intermittently.
4. In the oven, cook in a covered casserole dish for about 1 1/2-2 hours, more or less, or until the chicken is soft.

Indonesian Plaice

serves 1

- 1 Fillet of Plaice/Cod or other fish
- Black pepper
- Grated ginger root or ginger powder
- Pressed fresh garlic
- Chopped spring onions
- Olive oil

1. Lace the frying pan or dish with olive oil.
2. Place all the vegetables on the bottom and gently saute, whilst stirring.
3. When beginning to cook, place fish on top.
4. Put the lid on the pan and allow to cook through, adding a little water if food is sticking to the pan.
5. Check continuously and turn the fish if necessary.
6. Cook for 15 mins or until the fish is properly cooked through.

Note: This dish could also be baked in an oven in a covered dish for 1 hour or until cooked through.

Puddings

Exotic Coconut Pudding

- 1 tin coconut milk
- 2 bananas
- 1 large tin of pears in fruit juice (unsweetened.) Drain off liquid
- 1 passion fruit

1. Blend all the ingredients in the food processor until a creamy consistency is reached.
2. Serve chilled in dessert dishes over a pear or on its own. May be decorated with other fruit. If a thicker consistency is required, use less coconut milk.

This recipe can also be turned into ice-cream in an ice-cream maker.

Strawberries, Peaches Or Other Fruits With Cream

Pour single cream over the fruits of choice, e.g. washed strawberries sprinkled with fructose (fruit sugar), peaches or pears (tinned, sweetened with fruit juice), other berries or fruit salad.

Special Treats

Festive Birthday Cake

- 6 ozs bittersweet or semi-sweet chocolate melted over hot water and cooled *or* preferably use plain chocolate sweetened with fructose available from health shops or delicatessens
- 10 eggs separated and at room temperature
- 10 Tbsps (about 2/3 cup) fructose
- 2 cups finely chopped walnuts (not ground)

1. Preheat oven to 350 degrees F.
2. Beat the egg yolks and sugar until very thick and lemon coloured. Stir in the chocolate and fold in the nuts.
3. Beat the egg whites until stiff but not dry and fold into the chocolate-nut mixture. Turn in a greased 10 inch spring form pan and bake for 1 hour or until the centre springs back when lightly touched with the fingertips. Cool in the pan.

A variant could be to use finely grated carrots in place of chocolate.

Mouthwatering Gluten Free Chocolate-Chip Cookies (46)

- 200 grams butter
- 1 1/2 cups brown sugar OR 3/4 cup fructose
- 2 eggs
- 2 tsp vanilla essence
- 1 3/4 cups rice flour
- 1/4 cup buckwheat flour
- 1/4cup millet flakes
- 2 cups chocolate chips
- 1 cup chopped almonds
- 1 cup dessicated coconut
- 1 tsp baking soda-bicarb.
- (optional)

Note: try to bake these biscuits without the soda-bicarb. If absolutely necessary, use the minimum amount.

1. Cream butter, sugar, vanilla, eggs.
2. Add the dry ingredients and mix thoroughly.
3. Add choc chips, almonds, coconut and mix.
4. Form into cookies and bake on a greased baking tray for about 10 minutes at 190C.

2.10. Nutrient Content of Basic Foods

Calories, Quantity and Quality of Food

An adult usually needs at least 1,500 calories daily in order to maintain adequate energy and weight.

However, in this book the emphasis is on the frequency of ingesting *quality* foods which include the macro-nutrients carbohydrates, fats and proteins together with vitamins, minerals and essential fatty acids.

It is to be hoped that this approach will automatically provide a balanced diet with adequate calories. However, should weight control remain a problem - either too much or too little weight - it would be advisable to check the calorie intake daily, the absorption potential, as well as the physical exercise pattern with the relevant specialist. Even if there is no weight problem, exercise is an essential dimension to maintaining a healthy metabolism. Advice should be sought as to which type of exercise is suitable for the individual.

Some Good Food Sources of Nutrients *(48)*

N.B. Remember that foods which contain a high protein level can only be eaten at a specific time, when L-dopa medication is not relied upon.

Also, not all the foods are suitable for everyone, e.g. citrus, dairy foods or pulses might have to be excluded if indicated. Whole grains should also exclude gluten grains at all times for Parkinson's patients.

Carbohydrates
- Whole grains
- Honey
- Fruit
- Vegetables

Fats
- Butter and margarine
- Vegetable oils (cold pressed only)
- Nuts and seeds

Protein

- Fish and poultry
- Soybean
- Eggs
- Whole grains and Pulses

Water

- Mineral water
- Purified water
- Beverages
- Fruits
- Vegetables

Vitamin A and beta-carotene

- Liver (provided organic)
- Eggs
- Yellow fruits and vegetables
- Dark-green fruits and vegetables
- Whole milk and milk products

Vitamin B1

- Brewer's Yeast
- Whole grains
- Blackstrap molasses
- Brown rice
- Fish
- Poultry
- Egg yolks
- Legumes
- Nuts (not peanuts, cashews or brazils)

Vitamin B2

- Brewer's yeast
- Whole grains
- Blackstrap molasses
- Egg yolks
- Legumes
- Nuts

Vitamin B3 (Niacin)

- Brewer's yeast
- Poultry
- Fish
- Whole grains
- Milk products
- Rice Bran

Vitamin B5 (Pantothenic Acid)

- Brewer's yeast
- Egg yolks
- Legumes
- Whole grains
- Salmon

Vitamin B6

- Whole grains
- Brewer's yeast
- Blackstrap molasses
- Legumes
- Green leafy vegetables

Vitamin B12

- Fish
- Eggs
- Cheese
- Milk and Milk Products
- Unprocessed spirulina (B12 supplements advised for vegetarians)

Biotin

- Egg yolks
- Liver (organic)
- Unpolished rice
- Brewer's yeast
- Whole grains
- Sardines
- Legumes

Choline

- Egg yolks
- Brewer's yeast
- Soy Beans
- Fish
- Legumes

Folic Acid

- Dark green leafy vegetables
- Brewer's yeast
- Root vegetables
- Whole grains
- Oysters, Salmon, Milk

Inositol

- Whole grains
- Citrus fruits
- Brewer's yeast
- Molasses
- Milk
- Nuts (no peanuts, cashews and brazils)
- Vegetables

Para-Aminobenzoic Acid (PABA)

- Yoghurt
- Molasses
- Green leafy vegetables

Pantothenic Acid

- Brewer's yeast
- Egg yolks
- Legumes
- Whole grains
- Salmon

Vitamin C

- Citrus fruits
- Rose hips
- Acerola cherries
- Cantaloupe
- Strawberries
- Broccoli
- Tomatoes
- Green peppers

Vitamin D
- Salmon
- Sardines
- Herring
- Egg yolks

Vitamin E
- Cold pressed oils
- Eggs
- Molasses
- Sweet potatoes, leafy vegetables

Vitamin K
- Cauliflower
- Green leafy vegetables
- Egg yolks
- Safflower oil
- Blackstrap molasses
- Cauliflower
- Soy beans

Bioflavonoids
- Citrus fruits
- Fruits
- Blackcurrants
- Buckwheat

Unsaturated Fatty Acids
- Vegetable oils (cold pressed)
- Seeds (e.g. sunflower, sesame, pumpkin)

Calcium
- Milk
- Sesame seeds (Tahini) - extremely high content comparable with milk
- Green leafy vegetables
- Shellfish
- Molasses
- Sesame seeds (Tahini) - extremely high content comparable with milk

Chlorine
- Seafood
- Ripe olives

Chromium
- Honey
- Grapes
- Raisins
- Corn oil (cold pressed)
- Clams
- Whole grain cereals
- Brewer's yeast

Cobalt
- Oysters
- Clams
- Poultry
- Milk
- Green leafy vegetables
- Fruits

Copper
- Seafood
- Nuts
- Legumes
- Molasses
- Raisins

Fluoride
- Seafood

Iodine
- Seafood
- Kelp

Iron
- Eggs
- Fish
- Poultry
- Blackstrap molasses
- Cherry juice
- Green leafy vegetables
- Dried fruits
- Liver (organic)

Magnesium
- Seafood
- Whole grains
- Dark green vegetables
- Molasses
- Nuts and seeds

Manganese
- Whole grains
- Green leafy vegetables
- Legumes
- Nuts
- Pineapples
- Egg yolks

Molybdenum
- Legumes
- Whole-grain cereals
- Milk
- Kidney
- Liver (organic)
- Dark green vegetables

Phosphorous
- Fish
- Poultry
- Eggs
- Legumes
- Milk and Milk Products
- Nuts
- Whole grain cereals

Potassium
- Whole grains
- Vegetables
- Dried fruits
- Bananas
- Legumes
- Sunflower seeds

Selenium

- Tuna
- Herring
- Brewer's yeast
- Whole grains
- Sesame seeds

Sodium

- Seafood
- Celery

Sulphur

- Fish
- Garlic
- Onions
- Eggs
- Cabbage
- Brussels Sprouts
- Horseradish

Vanadium

- Fish

Zinc

- Pumpkin seeds
- Sunflower seeds
- Sesame seeds
- Seafood
- Oysters
- Mushrooms
- Brewer's yeast
- Herring
- Eggs

2.11. Some Approximate Food Values - Macronutrients and Calories of Key Carbohydrates, Proteins and Fats (49)

Carbohydrates

Brown Rice

Measure	1 cup
Weight	196 grams
Calories	704
Carbohydrate	152
Protein	14.8
Total Lipid	3.6

Rice Flour

Measure	1 cup
Weight	125 grams
Calories	479
Carbohydrate	107
Protein	7.5
Total Lipid	0.4

Millet Flour

Measure	1 cup
Weight	30 grams
Calories	100
Carbohydrate	21
Protein	3
Total lipid	1

Millet Flakes

Measure	1 cup
Weight	30 grams
Calories	100
Carbohydrate	21
Protein	3
Total lipids	1

Buckwheat Flour

Measure	1 cup
Weight	100 grams
Calories	333
Carbohydrate	72
Protein	11.7
Total lipids	2.5

Carob Flour

Weight	8 grams
Calories	14
Carbohydrates	6.5
Protein	0.4
Total lipids	0.1

Quinoa

Measure	1 cup
Weight	100 grams
Calories	335
Carbohydrates	59.9
Protein	14.9
Total lipids	5.8

Pumpkin

Measure	1 cup
Weight	245 grams
Calories	49
Carbohydrates	12
Protein	1.76
Total lipids	.17

Yams

Measure	1 cup
Weight	200
Calories	210
Carbohydrates	48.2
Protein	4.8
Total lipids	0.4

Plantain

Weight	100 grams
Calories	112
Carbohydrates	28.5
Protein	0.8
Total lipids	0.2

Sweet Potato

Weight	100 grams
Calories	87
Carbohydrates	21.3
Protein	1.2
Total Lipids	0.3

Proteins

Soy Beans (cooked)

Measure	1 cup
Weight	180 grams
Calories	234
Carbohydrates	19.4
Protein	19.8
Total lipids	10.3
Total unsaturated	7.68
Cholesterol	Nil

Raw green peas

Measure	100 grams
Carbohydrate	10
Protein	6
Total lipids	1.6

Chicken (light meat)

Measure	4 ozs
Weight	116 grams
Calories	216
Carbohydrate	Nil
Protein	23.5
Total lipids	12.8
Total unsaturated	7.96
Cholesterol	78

Turkey (light meat)

Measure	6.4 ozs
Weight	180 grams
Calories	286
Carbohydrate	Nil
Protein	39
Total lipids	13.2
Total unsaturated	8.18
Cholesterol	117

Fish (cod)

Measure	3 ozs
Weight	85 grams
Calories	70
Carbohydrate	Nil
Protein	15
Total lipids	0.57
Total unsaturates	0.276
Cholesterol	37

Eggs (whole)

Measure	1 large
Weight	50 grams
Calories	79
Carbohydrates	0.6
Protein	6.07
Total lipids	5.58
Total unsaturates	2.97
Cholesterol	274

Baker's Yeast (dried)

Weight	100 grams
Calories	169
Carbohydrates	3.5
Protein	35.6
Total Lipids	1.5

Fats

Almonds

Measure	1 cup
Weight	142 grams
Calories	849
Carbohydrates	27.7
Protein	26.4
Total lipids	77
Total unsaturated	67
Cholesterol	Nil

Sesame Seeds

Measure	1 cup
Weight	150 grams
Calories	873
Carbohydrates	26.4
Protein	27.3
Total lipids	80
Total unsaturated	64
Cholesterol	Nil

Coconut - Desiccated

Weight	100 grams
Calories	604
Carbohydrates	6.4
Protein	5.6
Total lipids	62
Total unsaturated	1.5
Saturated	4.7
Monounsaturated	50
Cholesterol	Nil

Olive Oil

Measure	1 tablespoon
Weight	13.5 grams
Calories	119
Carbohydrates	Nil
Protein	Nil
Total lipids	13.5
Total Unsaturated	11
Cholesterol	Nil

Butter

Measure	1 tble spoon
Weight	14.1
Calories	101
Carbohydrates	.008
Protein	0.12
Total lipids	11.5
Total Unsaturated	3.74
Cholesterol	31

Light Whipping Cream

Measure	1 cup
Weight	239 grams
Calories	699
Protein	5.15
Carbohydrates	7.07
Total lipids	73.8
Total unsaturated	23.8
Cholesterol	265

APPENDIX

3.1. GLOSSARY OF TERMS

(NB this glossary has been prepared to give the meaning of terms as used in this book, not to give their complete definition in any other context.)

Absorption site - area of the digestive system where a specific nutrient is absorbed through the gut wall.

Acetyl choline - an important neurotransmitter - also called a transmitter substance - liberated at synapses in the central nervous system, that stimulates skeletal muscle contraction.

Active transport - absorption of a substance against the concentration gradient, using energy.

Adrenal medulla - the inner portion of the adrenal gland which secretes epinephrine and norepinephrine (adrenaline and noradrenaline.)

Agonist - a drug which upon binding to a receptor on the pre or post synaptic membrane produces a response similar to that caused by the neurotransmitter released at the synapse.

Alkaline foods - those which leave an alkaline residue in the body, including most fruit and vegetables, some grains and seeds.

Amino acids - smallest building blocks of protein, produced during digestion.

Anabolism - energy requiring reactions, where small molecules are built up into larger ones.

Antioxidant - enzyme or nutrient which neutralises a damaging free radical.

Appropriate fibre - in this case meaning fibre foods 'containing no gluten'.

ATP - adenosine tri-phosphate - the universal energy carrying molecule, which is formed during energy releasing reactions in the Kreb's Cycle.

Autogenic training - a technique taught by psychologists to aid in the control of stress.

Bifidobacteria - a group of healthy bacteria found in the normal gut.

Bio-feedback - in this sense a psychology technique to aid in the control of stress.-

Biosynthesis - the manufacture of complex substances within the body.

Blood-brain barrier - a barrier of special capillaries which controls the passage of substances into the brain and its fluid.

91

Carbohydrate loading - in this sense, regularly imbibing carbohydrate ensuring a constant supply of glucose for the brain.

Cell- the smallest unit of biological activity, in which metabolic processes take place.

Chelation - use of certain organic molecules which bond with toxic metals and aid their removal from the body.

Co-enzyme - an organic molecule which activates an enzyme: many are derived from vitamins.

Co-factor - substance which combines with the protein part of an enzyme and activates it: it may be a metal ion, eg zinc, iron, or a co-enzyme.

Competition for absorption - the digestive system has specific areas for absorption of various nutrients and different substances may compete for absorption there. Different substances may also compete for the same transport mechanisms.

Dopamine - a neurotransmitter active in certain areas of the brain and involved in certain movements of skeletal muscles.

Dysbiosis - abnormal and unhealthy changes in the balance of bacteria and other micro-organisms present in the gut.

Dyskinesia - abnormality of motor function characterized by involuntary, purposeless movements.

EPA, ecosapentanoic acid - an important fatty acid with 5 double bonds; it is used in the body to make anti-inflammatory prostaglandins.

Fatty acid - a carbon chain with hydrogen atoms attached to the carbon; it is normally found in food as a triglyceride, with three fatty acids attached to a glycerol molecule.

Free form - individual small molecules (eg amino acids), which are not any longer combined as in their normal form (eg whole proteins.) They are ready to be absorbed.

Free radical - an unstable molecular fragment with an unpaired electron which is looking for a 'partner' electron, which it can steal from other molecules, damaging them.

Fructose - the simple sugar found in most fruit; it has to be converted into glucose before use as an energy source, slowing its activity down.

GLA, gama linolenic acid - an important fatty acid made in healthy cells, and also found in certain seed oils, eg evening primrose and borage.

Glucose loading - see carbohydrate loading.

Glucose tolerance factor - a substance containing chromium and vitamin B3 which works with insulin to facilitate glucose entry to cells.

Gluten - a sticky protein found in wheat, oats, barley, rye and spelt which may possibly reduce absorption through the gut wall; it causes major damage to the intestinal wall in coeliac disease.

Glycaemic pattern - carbohydrate metabolism.

Glycaemic pathway - carbohydrate metabolism.

Guar gum - a soluble fibre which may be supplemented to increase bulk and to slow glucose absorption.

Gut flora - the total population of bacteria and other micro-organisms in the gut.

Helicobacter pylori - a bacterium which can survive the acid conditions in the stomach; it may lead to gastritis, ulcer and even stomach cancer.

Hydrogenated - a commercial process whereby the double bonds in unsaturated fatty acids have extra hydrogen added, in fact making them saturated.

Hyperpermeable gut - increased permeability of the gut wall which allows entry of large molecules, eg undigested protein, into the blood stream which can stimulate an allergic reaction. Tests exist to determine the degree of permeability.

Integrity of the gut lining - refers to fully functional cell membranes or epithelium lining the gut, which can control absorption of nutrients or other substances.

Hypoglycaemic state - below normal concentration of glucose in the blood, producing specific symptoms.

Intoxication - toxic effect of chemicals on cell function, including not only alcohol and other drugs, but also toxic metals, nerve gas, sprays and many food additives etc.

Kreb's cycle (citric acid cycle) - a series of energy releasing chemical reactions in the mitochondria of cells.

L-dopa - abbreviation for levodopa.

Levadopa - L-dopa, the synthetic pharmaceutical medication which replaces the natural substance normally produced in cells but which is lacking in Parkinson's patients.

Lactobacillus acidophilus - a bacterium found naturally in the healthy gut and in good probiotic supplements.

Long chain polymer - a large molecule made up of a chain of similar small molecules, eg starch is a polymer of glucose.

Melanin - the dark pigment found in skin, and increased in suntan.

Metabolism - the sum of the chemical reactions which take place in cells.

93

Mitochondria - small organelles within each cell where energy is released for use in cell activity.

NADH - The name of the product NADH is the abbreviation for the reduced form of nicotinamide-adenine-dinucleotide. This reduced form contains high-energy hydrogen (the H in NADH) that provides energy to the cell. Nicotinamide is a form of vitamin B3. The NADH supplement assists the energy production in all cells.

Naso-gastric tube - tubing carrying liquid food from its source via the nose.

Neurone - a nerve cell, with long processes which carry the nerve impulse.

Neurotoxin - a toxin which can affect the function of the nervous system.

Neurotransmitter - a chemical which transmits the nerve impulse from one neurone to the next.

Neutral amino acids - specific essential amino acids contained in protein.

Noradrenalin - a hormone similar to adrenalin.

Omega 3 fatty acid - a family of essential fatty acids, mainly obtained from cold water fish, and also flax seed oil, used to form anti-inflammatory prostaglandins.

Omega 6 fatty acid - a family of esential fatty acids found in evening primrose oil, borage and other seed oils, which can form either pro- or anti-inflammatory prostaglandins.

Orthomolecular - literally 'the right molecule' - usually as in treatment of disease using the optimum amount of nutrients.

Pallidotomy - brain operation which is implicated in the control of tremor.

Parenteral - via the vein.

Peripheral decarboxylase inhibitor - a substance which prevents the premature breakdown of L-dopa and thus enables it to penetrate the Blood Brain Barrier in optimum form.

Peristalsis - successive muscular contractions along the wall of the gut, which moves food or waste products.

Permeability - the size of openings in the gut wall which affects entry of different sized molecules.

pH - symbol indicating how acid or alkaline a substance is: below 7 is acid, 7 is neutral, above 7 is alkaline.

Precursor - a substance which is converted into another substance in the body.

Probiotics - encouraging healthy bacteria in the gut, usually by supplementing, eg Lactobacillus acidophilus and Bifidobacteria, to improve the immunity and health of the gut and also of the rest of the body.

Prostaglandins - fatty acids converted in the body to perform specific hormone-like functions in regulation of cell activity.

Protease - enzyme which digests protein.

Protein window - in this book used to describe the time period when concentrated protein may be eaten - when L-dopa medication is not needed.

Striatum - corpus striatum - an area in the interior of each cerebral hemisphere of the brain.

Sublingual - absorption of a supplement under the tongue.

Substantia nigra - a large nucleus in the mid brain, considered part of the basal ganglia and containing dopamine producing neurones.

Synthesis - chemical reactions manufacturing complex substances from simple ones.

Transdermal - absorption of a substance through the skin.

Trans fats - fatty acids which have been damaged in processing, and can no longer be used by the body. They may block reactions using essential fatty acids.

Transit time - time it takes for food to be digested and the indigestible residue eliminated.

Unhydrogenated - natural fatty acids, which have not been processed with hydrogen to make them solid.

Vasodilation - expansion in the diameter of a blood vessel.

Vesicles - membraneous sacs within cells, which transport substances into, across or out of the cell.

3.2. REFERENCES

1. Dietary Factors in the Management of Parkinson's Disease: P.A. Kempster, MD MRCP FRACP, M.C.Wahlqvist MD FRACP, Nutrition Reviews Vol 52, No. 2, 1994

2. Janice Fuller, B.Pharm., Du Pont Pharmaceuticals Ltd., Avenue One, Letchworth Garden City, Hertfordshire, SG6 2HU, England

3. Biochemistry: The National Medical series for Independent Study, 1994, p.476: Victor L Davidson, Ph D, Donald B Sittman, Ph D, Harwal Publishing, A Waverly Company, Baltimore, United States of America

4. Optimum Nutrition Workbook: Patrick Holford, B.Sc., Dip ION: 1992: p 34: ION Press,Blades Court, Deodar Road, London SW15 2NU

5. op.cit. n.3 p.371

6. Wills' Biochemical Basis of Medicine. J. Hywel Thomas, PhD. & Brian Gillham PhD., pps 417, 418, published by Butterworth Heinemann Limited, 1993, Linacre House, Jordan Hill, Oxford OX2 8DP, England

7. op.cit. n.6

8. op.cit. n.1

9. Hospital Update: Book Review: Artificial Nutrition Support in Clinical Practice: August 1995: Hayes Peter

10. Acta Neurologica Scandinavia: 1993: 87: Suppl.146: 32-35: J.Birkmeyer

11. op.cit. n.10

12. Motor Effects of Broad Beans (Vicia Faba) in Parkinson's Disease: Single Dose Studies: P.A.Kempster MD et al: 1993: Asia Pacific Journal of Nutrition,2, 85-89:

13. BioLab Medical Unit, The Stone House, 9 Weymouth Street, London W1N 3FF: IgG Tests (ELIZA) are available through Higher Nature Ltd., Burwash Common, East Sussex TN19 7LX, England

14. ABPI Data Sheet Compendium: 1994-1995: See Sinemet and Madopar

15. The Lactic Acid Bacteria - their Role in Human Health: Dr Nigel Plummer: 1992: Biomed Publications Limited, Westminster House, 189-190 Stratford House, Shirley, West Midlands, England B90 3AQ

16. ProBiotics: Leon Chaitow, N.D., D.O., and Natasha Trenev: 1990: Thorsons, Harper Collins Publishers, 77-85 Fulham Palace Road, Hammersmith, London W6 8JB

17. Parkinson's Disease. Dr Abraham N. Lieberman and Frank Williams: 1993 Balance of Transmitters, p 35. Thorsons, 77-85 Fulham Palace Road, Hammersmith, London W6 8JB

18. Nutrition Almanac: (p 228): Lavon J. Dunne: 1990: Mc-Graw Hill Publishing Company, New York

19. Wills' Biochemical Basis of Medicine: Second Edition: 1993 (p 417). J. Hywel Thomas, PhD, F.I.Biol, & Brian Gillham, PhD: Butterworth-Heinemann Ltd., Linacre House, Jordan Hill, Oxford OX2 8DP

20. op.cit. n.4

21. Nutrition Reviews, Volume 52, No 2, p. 54: Dietary Factors in The Management of Parkinson's Disease: P.A. Kempster M D MRCP FRACP and M.L. Wahlqvist M D FRACP

22. Wills' Biochemical Basis of Medicine: Second Edition, 1993: (p426): J. Hywel Thomas, PhD., FIBiol & Brian Gillham PhD., (p 426): Published by Butterworth Heinemann Limited, Linacre House, Jordan Hill, Oxford OX2 8DP.

23. op.cit. n.12

24. op.cit. n.10

25. op.cit. n.10

26. op.cit. n.2

27. Nutrition Reviews, Volume 52, No 2, p. 52: Dietary Factors in The Management of Parkinson's Disease: P.A. Kempster M D MRCP FRACP and M.L. Wahlqvist M D FRACP

28. Optimum Nutrition Workbook: Patrick Holford:, B.Sc., Dip ION. 1992: p.148: ION Press, Blades Court, Deodar Road, London SW15 2NU

29. Konjac Fibre is manufactured by Health Plus Limited, PO Box 86, Seaford, East Sussex, BN25 4ZW, England

30. op.cit. n.21

31. Nutrition Almanac: Lavon J. Dunne: 1990 Nutrition Search Inc., McGraw Hill, New York, U.S.A.

32. The Composition of Foods: McCance and Widowson: 1993: The Royal Society of Chemistry, Thomas Graham House, Science Park, Milton Road, Cambridge CB4 4WF, U.K., and the Ministry of Agriculture, Fisheries and Food.

33. How to Improve your Digestion and Absorption: Christopher Scarfe: 1988. p14: ION Press, Blades Court, Deodar Road, London SW15 2NU.

34. New Facts about Fiber: Betty Kaman, PhD: 1991: p15: Nutrition Encounter Inc., Box 2736, Novato, California 94948, U.S..

35. Fibre and Bulk Preparations: K.W. Heaton: 1991: pps 212,213. Extract from Gastrointestinal Transit (Pathophysiology and Pharmacology): Wrightson Biomedical Publishing Ltd., Ash Barn House, Winchester Road, Stroud, Petersfield, Hampshire GU3 2PN, England.

36. Better Health through Natural Healing: Ross Trattler, N.D., D.O., 1987: p191: Thorsons Publishers Limited, Wellingborough, Northamptonshire, NN8 2RQ, England

37. Better Health through Natural Healing: Ross Trattler, N.D., D.O.: 1987: p190: Thorsons Publishers Limited, Wellingborough, Northamptonshire, NN8 2RQ, England

38. New Facts about Fiber: Betty Kaman, PhD: 1991: pps 19 & 59: Nutrition Encounter Inc., Box 2736, Novato, California 94948, U.S..A.

39. Parkinson's Disease: Dr. Abraham N. Lieberman & Frank Williams, 1993. P 154. Thorsons, 77-85 Fulham Palace Road, London W6 8JB

40. op.cit. n.15

41. ABPI Data Sheet Compendium: 1994-1995: see Flagyl (p1248): Datapharm Publications Limited, 12 Whitehall, London SW1A 2DY

42. op.cit. n.43

43. Fats that Heal: Fats that Kill: Udo Erasmus: 1993: pps 110,111: Alive Books, 7436 Frazer Park Drive, Burnaby B.C., Canada V5J 5B

44. The Clinical Science of Mineral Therapy: Dr Leslie Fisher: 1993: pps 39 & 40.

45. Beat Candida Cookbook: Erica White, Dip. ION: 1992: p78: 22 Leigh Hall Road, Leigh-on-Sea, Essex SS9 1RN

46. Janice Trachtman: 1996.

47. Karen Segal: 1996.

48. Nutrition Almanac, 3rd Edition: Lavon J. Dunne, Nutrition Search Inc: 1990: McGraw Hill, New York, U.S.A.

49. op.cit. n.48

3.3. BIBLIOGRAPHY

Biochemistry: The National Medical Series for Independent Study, 1994, Victor L Davidson, Ph D, Donald B Sittman, Ph D, Harwal Publishing, A Waverly Company, Baltimore, United States of America.

Wills' Biochemical Basis of Medicine: Second Edition, 1993 J. Hywel Thomas, PhD., FIBiol & Brian Gillham PhD., (p 426): Published by Butterworth Heinemann Limited, Linacre House, Jordan Hill, Oxford OX2 8DP.

Nutrition Almanac, 3rd Edition: Lavon J. Dunne, Nutrition Search Inc: 1990: McGraw Hill, New York, U.S.A.

The Composition of Foods, 5th Edition: McCance and Widowson: 1993: published by The Royal Society of Chemistry, Thomas Graham House, Science Park, Milton Road, Cambridge CB4 4WF, U.K., and The Ministry of Agriculture, Fisheries and Food.

Gastrointestinal Transit (Pathophysiology and Pharmacology): 1991: edited by Michael A. Kamm and John E. Lennard-Jones: Wrightson Biomedical Publishing Ltd., Ash Barn House, Winchester Road, Stroud, Petersfield, Hampshire

Parkinson's Disease: Dr Abraham N. Lieberman and Frank Williams: 1993: Thorsons, An Imprint of Harper Collins Publishers, 77-85 Fulham Palace Road, Hammersmith, London W6 8JB.

Principles of Anatomy and Physiology, 6th Edition, 1990: Gerard J. Tortora & Nicholas P. Anagnostakos. Published by Harper Collins Publishers, 10 East 53rd Street, New York, N.Y. 10022, U.S.A.

Textbook of Medical Physiology: Arthur C. Guyton, M.D.: 5th edition 1976: W.B. Saunders Company, West Washington Square, Philadelphia, PA 19105, U.S.A.

Clinical Medicine, edited by Parveen J. Kumar and Micheal L. Clark, 3rd printing: 1992: Bailliere Tindall, 24-28 Oval Road, London NW1 7DX

The Merck Manual, 16th Edition, 1992: edited by Robert Berkow, M.D. and Andrew J. Fletcher, M.B., B. Chir: Merck Research Laboratories, Division of Merck & Co., Inc., Rahway, N.J., U.S.A.

Analysis of the Effects of the Removal of Gluten and other unknown Compounds contained in Wheat and Gluten Grains, Rye, Oats and Barley in Sufferers of the Irritable Bowel Syndrome: Lucille Leader: 1994: Research Project: Institute for Optimum Nutrition, London (Supervisor, Dr Philip Barlow, MSc. PhD., Associate Dean, School of Food Studies, University of Humberside, Hull., U.K.. and Supervisor of Research Studies, Institute for Optimum Nutrition, London)

Nutritional Medicine: Dr Stephen Davies, B.Sc., M.B., Ch.B and Dr Alan Stewart, M.B., ChB., MRCP; 1987: published by Pan Books Limited, Cavaye Place, London SW10 9PG

Dietary Factors in the Management of Parkinson's Disease: P.A. Kempster, M.D., M R.C.P. (U.K.), F.R.A.C.P. and Prof. M.L. Wahlqvist, M.D., F.R.A.C.P.: Nutrition Reviews, Vo. 52, No. 2, February 1994: Dr Kempster is with the Department of Neurosciences and Medicine and Dr Wahlqvist is with the Department of Medicine, Monash Medical Centre, 246 Clayton Road, Clayton 3168, Melbourne, Australia

Supplements for Parkinson's Disease: Pat Lazarus: Let's Live: July 1992. (Author's Note: For a list of orthomolecular physicians, contact the Huxley Institute, 900 North Federal Highway, Suite 330, Boca Raton, FL33432, USA or call 407/393-6167)

The Amino Revolution - Dr Robert Erdman, Ph.D. and Meirion Jones 1987 - published by Century Hutchinson Limited, Brookmount, 62-65 Chandos Place, Covent Garden, London WC2N 4NW

Thorsons Guide to Amino Acids - Leon Chaitow N.D.D.O. - 1991 - published by Thorsons, 77-85 Fulham Palace Road, London W6 8JB

The Healing Nutrients Within (Facts, Findings and New Research on Amino Acids: 1987: Eric R. Braverman, M.D., with Carl C. Pfeiffer, M.D., Ph.D. Keats Publishing Inc, 27 Pine Street (B.K.), New Canaan, Connecticut, U.S.A.

Mental and Elemental Nutrients, Carl C. Pfeiffer, M.D., Ph.D. (and the publications committee of the Brain Biocentre, Princeton, New Jersey), 1975: Keats Publishing Inc., 27 Pine Street (B.K.) New Canaan, Connecticut 06840, U.S.A.

Better Health through Natural Healing: Ross Trattler, M.D., D.O.: 1987: Thorsons Publishers Limited, Wellingborough, Northamptonshire, NN8 2RQ, U.K.

Diet and Nutrition: Rudolph Ballantine, M.D.: 1989: published by the Himalayan International Institute, Box 400, Homesdale, Pennsylvania 18431, U.S..

Minerals - the Metabolic Miracle Workers: Dr Robert Erdman, Ph.D. and Meirion Jones: 1988: Century Hutchinson, Brookmount House, 62-65 Chandos Place, Covent Garden, London WC2N 4NW

The Lactic Acid Bacteria - their Role in Human Health: 1992: Dr Nigel Plummer, B.Sc., PhD: BioMed Publications Limited, Westminster House, 189-190 Stratford Road, Shirley, West Midlands B90 3AQ, U.K.

Optimum Nutrition Workbook: Patrick Holford: 2nd, Revised Edition 1992: ION Press, 5 Jerdan Place, London SW6 1BE, U.K.

Super Foods: Michael van Straten and Barbara Griggs: reprinted 1993: Dorling Kindersley Limited, 9 Henrietta Street, London WC2E 8PS

Characterisation of the In Vivo Behaviour of a Controlled-Release Formulation of Levodopa (Sinemet CR): 1991: I.R. Wilding, J.G. Hardy, S.S. Davis, C.D. Melia, D.F. Evans, A.H. Short, R.A. Sparrow, K.C. yeh: Clinical Neuropharmacology, Vol. 14, No. 4, pp 305-321: Raven Press Ltd., New York. Address correspondence and reprint requests to: Dr I.R. Wilding at Pharmaceutical Profiles Limited, 2 Faraday Building, Highfields Science Park, University Boulevard, Nottingham NG7 2QP, U.K.

First Emergence of "Delayed-On" and "Dose Failure" Phenomena in a Patient with Parkinson's Disease following Vagotomy: Ruth Djaldetti, Anat Achiron, Ilan Ziv, Eldad Melamed, Department of Neurology, Beilinson Medical Center and the Felsenstein Research Institute, Petah Tiqva, Israel: Movement Disorders, Vol. 9, No. 5, 1994, pp 582-583

Magic Beans? Natural Sources of L-dopa in the treatment of Parkinson's Disease: Dan Beth-El: International Journal of Alternative and Complementary Medicine, September 1992

Motor Effects of Broad Beans(Vicia faba) in Parkinson's Disease: Single dose studies: P.A. Kempster MD et al: Depts. of Neurosciences, Medicine and Biochemistry, Monash Medical Centre, Melbourne, Australia: Asia Pacific Journal of Clinical Nutrition:1993, 2, 85-89

3.4. INDEX

A

Absorption, 25, 43, 91, 98
Acetylcholine, 12, 14, 43
Adrenal medulla, 91
Alcohol, 23, 51, 76
Alkaline, 91
Almonds, 22, 28, 51, 87
Amino acids, 14, 91
anabolic function, 3
Antioxidants, 17
Apple, 56, 74, 75

B

Banana, 75
Barley, 4, 100
Bifido bacteria, 4, 12
Birkmeyer, 10, 17, 96
Blood, 24, 91, 94
Bowel, 4, 100
Buckwheat, 25, 53, 82, 85
Butter, 21, 26, 47, 50, 54, 57, 68, 70, 74, 79, 87

C

Calcium, 16, 82
Camomile, 25
Carbohydrate, 39, 85, 86, 92
Carbohydrate loading, 39, 92
Cheese, 81
Chicken, 28, 34, 76, 86
Chicory, 26, 57
Coconut, 54, 77, 87
Coffee, 23, 26, 51, 57
Constipation, 29, 31, 32, 45
Corn, 25, 47, 53, 57, 82
Cutlery, 36

D

Dairy, 21, 28
Dandelion, 26
Dentist, 36
Depression, 35, 45
Diet, 13, 34, 46, 48, 101
Digestive enzyme, 10, 12
Dopamine, 1, 14, 16, 43, 92
Dyskinesia, 92

E

Egg, 80, 81, 82, 83
Energy, 27, 44
Enzymes, 17, 43
Essential fatty acids, 2, 4, 9
Exercise, 29, 33, 35

F

Fibre, 4, 24, 29, 34, 45, 97, 98
Fish, 28, 34, 80, 81, 83, 84, 86
Flours, 26
Fluids, 29
Fruits, 13, 34, 77, 80, 82

G

Gluten, 4, 26, 28, 47, 53, 55, 56, 65, 71, 72, 73, 78, 93, 100
Glycaemic, 93
Grains, 4, 21, 25, 100
Gut flora, 93

H

Herb teas, 57
Hippocrates, 5
Hypoglycaemic, 93

L

Levodopa, 25, 39, 101

M

Madopar, 12, 19, 96
Magnesium, 83
Maize, 25, 53
Margarine, 26, 50, 57
Microwave, 70
Milk, 21, 27, 34, 80, 81, 82, 83
Millet, 25, 53, 66, 85
Minerals, 11, 12, 16, 101
Music, 35

N

NAD, 17
NADH, 3, 9, 10, 12, 17, 94
Neurotoxin, 94
Nuts, 22, 34, 50, 79, 80, 81, 83

O

Olive oil, 70, 73, 77

P

Pastas, 53, 56
Phenylalanine, 14
Physiotherapy, 33
Plantains, 50, 53
Protein, 9, 20, 28, 37, 39, 50, 54, 65, 76, 80, 85, 86, 87, 95
Psychologist, 35
Pulses, 21, 22, 25, 28, 51, 80
Pumpkin seeds, 84

Q

Quinoa, 25, 85

R

Recipes, 20, 26, 60, 65, 76
Rice crackers, 53

S

Salad, 63, 64, 70
Seeds, 22, 28, 34, 51, 82, 87
Sesame seeds, 82, 84
Sinemet, 12, 19, 96, 101
Soy, 81, 82, 86
Soya, 21, 22, 28, 44, 51, 54
Spinach, 28
Spreads, 26, 57
Stress, 11, 35, 45
Sugar, 24, 27
Sunflower seeds, 83, 84
Supplements, 11, 100

T

Tapioca, 25, 53
Tryptophan, 14
Tyrosine, 14, 16

V

Vegetables, 25, 79, 80, 81, 83
Vitamin, 3, 12, 16, 39, 80, 81, 82
Vitamins, 3, 11, 12, 16, 44

W

Wahlqvist, 5, 96, 97, 100
Water, 26, 46, 51, 80
Weight, 2, 85, 86, 87

Z

Zinc, 16, 84